25 STEPS TO SAFE COMPUTING

Peachpit Press

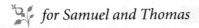 *for Samuel and Thomas*

25 STEPS TO SAFE COMPUTING
Don Sellers

PEACHPIT PRESS
2414 Sixth St.
Berkeley, CA 94710
(510) 548-4393
(510) 548-5991 (fax)

Find us on the World Wide Web at:
http://www.peachpit.com

Peachpit Press is a division of Addison-Wesley Publishing Company.

Copyright ©1995 Don Sellers
Interior design: Don Sellers
Cover design: TMA Ted Mader Associates

QUANTITY PURCHASES
This book and other Peachpit titles are available for quantity purchase. For more information contact Peachpit Press at (800) 980-8999 or (510) 548-5762.

ISBN 0-201-88366-X

0 9 8 7 6 5 4 3 2 1

Printed and bound in the United States of America

Printed on recycled paper.

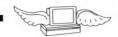

Acknowledgments

We thank these computer-health experts whose generosity with their time and knowledge made this book possible.

■ ■ ■

- Dennis Ankrum, Director of Human Factors Research, Nova Office Furniture
- Bruce Bernard, MD, MPH, National Institute of Occupational Safety and Health (NIOSH)
- Robert Bettendorf, Institute for Office Ergonomics
- Mark Caitlin, WASHCOSH
- Richard Cheu, Vision Aerobics
- Elizabeth Collumb, Voyager Company
- Paul Cornell, PhD, Steelcase, Inc.
- Andrea Devaux, American Academy of Ophthalmology
- Mary Flynn, OD, Illinois College of Optometry
- Fred Frietag, BO, Diamond Headache Clinic
- Janet Gold, Labor Occupational Health Center
- Chris Grant, PhD, University of Michigan
- Michelle Hartzell, NoRad Corp.
- Rob Henning, PhD, University of Connecticut
- Pamela Henwood, Visionary Software
- Peter Jeff, Steelcase, Inc.
- Pete Johnson, Ergonomics Laboratory at the University of California at Berkeley and San Francisco
- Marilyn Joyce, The Joyce Institute
- Jim Kinsella, *CTDNews*
- Ruth Lowengart, MD, Alta Bates Occupational Health Clinic
- Rani Lueder, Humanics
- Shirley Lunde, Kinesis Corporation
- Steve Marshall, The Ergonomics Lab
- Bob Matthews, Sonera Technologies
- Dennis McIntosh, Center for Office Technology
- Stephen C. Miller, OD, American Optometric Association
- Lori Parent, Curtis Manufacturing
- Vern Putz-Anderson, PhD, NIOSH
- Ward Raap, National EMF Testing Association
- David Rempel, MD, Ergonomics Laboratory at the University of California at Berkeley and San Francisco
- Scott Robinson, V.P. & Manager of Safety & Health, Wells Fargo Corp.
- Caroline Rose, RSI Network
- Hector Serber, American Ergonomics Corporation
- Dr. James Sheedy, VDT Eye Clinic, University of California
- Michael Silva, Enertech Consultants
- Louis Slesin, *VDT NEWS*
- Michael J. Smith, PhD, Department of Industrial Engineering, University of Wisconsin at Madison
- Suzanne Stefanac
- Debbie Stiles, MN, RN, Healthy Dimensions
- Laura Stock, Labor Occupational Health Program
- Naomi Swanson, PhD, NIOSH
- Susan Thomas, Signa Corporation
- Beverley Tillery, Office Technology Education Project
- Ignacio Valdes, LifeTime Software
- Thomas van Overbeek, Cornerstone Technology
- Tim Warner, *Macworld* Magazine
- Jim Young, NYCOSH

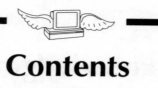

Contents

■ ■ ■

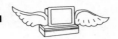

How to Read This Book

∎ ∎ ∎

For you to get the most out of this book, think of it as one of the tools at your disposal: the book supplies the information, but you must add your own intelligence and common sense. This book can act as your guide, but it cannot necessarily tell you exactly what you should do in any particular situation.

Don't Let It Replace a Doctor

To make this book useful for the largest number of people, we have included more information than most people need—so much, in fact, that you may have to steer clear of some. For example, should everyone perform the stretches and exercises on pages 26–27? Absolutely not: Sometimes illness or other factors make exercise a bad idea. We also describe how certain medical conditions are typically handled. Should you handle them that way? Perhaps. Only a health-care professional, and ultimately a physician, can tell you what is best for your body. Although this book includes the most up-to-date information from physicians, scientists, ergonomists, and other experts in the computer-health field, no book is capable of acting as a health-care professional.

Be a Low-Stress Reader

This book's tone expresses a calm and reasoned concern about the health issues involved in computer use. We made this choice for a good reason: Psychological stress may worsen many of the physical problems associated with computer use. Worry is counterproductive. Don't dwell on aspects of the job you can't change. Instead, read this book with a positive attitude, figure out what you need and can do, and then take action.

Be Involved

There's no way of ensuring that computer work will never hurt you. But you can take some of the simple steps included in this book to reduce your chances of injury. The key is that *you* must take the steps; no one else can take them for you. Most of the steps require very little effort. Browse through the book and try out some of the suggestions in the areas that catch your eye. Keep in mind that one change often leads to another. Taking responsibility for your own health will pay dividends in all areas of your life.

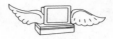

Introduction

■ ■ ■

Computer-related injuries have risen dramatically over the last few years. Bureau of Labor Statistics surveys show that in 1981, when the desktop computer was just being introduced, cumulative trauma disorders (CTDs) accounted for 18% of all workplace illnesses in the United States (this includes all industries, like meat packing and working in a super-market). By 1993, when there were over 50 million desktop computers in use, the figure had risen to over 62%. Recently, a *CTDNews* survey concluded that 4.4 million people in the United States suffer from computer-related CTDs.

The High Cost

No one knows how much this costs businesses, but most rough estimates place it in the tens of billions of dollars. The National Council on Compensation Insurance figures that treating a single case of back pain costs business about $24,000; treating a single case of carpal tunnel syndrome costs $29,000. The cost of the human suffering is harder to estimate. Most computer users don't know what can injure them. And people often work on computers until they are so injured that a return to good health proves difficult or impossible. People need a guide, which was our objective when we created *25 Steps to Safe Computing*.

The Handbook

25 Steps has its roots in another book, *Zap! How your computer can hurt you—and what you can do about it*, first published in 1994. Although *Zap!* was written to be an easily accessible handbook, we also made it comprehensive. People loved *Zap!* but told us they wanted something simpler, a quick reference to making computer work safer. We distilled and updated the contents of *Zap!* to create *25 Steps to Safe Computing*.

The Safe Attitude

But staying healthy requires more than a book sitting on your desk. Minimizing computer-related stress—both psychological and physical—requires a fundamental shift in attitude. The safe computing attitude requires you to act constructively *before* you feel the pain. One after another, major corporations have begun to nurture this attitude in their employees, making office safety a top priority, because better health pays benefits for everyone. It can for you, too.

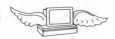

Your Office Is an Ecosystem
■ ■ ■

It may seem odd to regard your office as an ecosystem, but it is. Your workplace environment holds living, breathing organisms—you and your co-workers. The quality of your health results from a delicate balance between a combination of:

- What you bring with you to the office (how much you exercise, what you ate the night before, your outlook on life)
- The physical characteristics of the office (lighting, furniture, quality of the air)
- The requirements of your job (intensity of your keyboard use, amount of work rotation)
- The psychosocial aspects of the workplace (deadlines, attitude of your manager, the emphasis your company puts on health)

An Ecosystem in Trouble

Lately, many office ecosystems are experiencing increased stress coming from a variety of sources, including:

- The downsizing of many businesses
- Drives for increased productivity
- Inadequately designed equipment and furniture
- The rise in computer use

This stress can injure people. Computer-related injuries exact a high cost to employers and society due to medical treatment, lost wages, lost productivity, and retraining of disabled workers.

These injuries—most commonly involving the hands, wrists, arms, neck, and back—can be debilitating. The earlier they are diagnosed and correctly treated, the more likely the recovery to good health.

It's All Hooked Together

The interdependent nature of different elements in the office ecosystem makes intervention a challenge. When you act to achieve safety at your computer, you often discover that a change in one component affects others. For example, your wrists hurt, so you raise your chair to keep them flatter while typing. But then your legs start to hurt because your feet are no longer resting on the floor. Or you may find that your neck

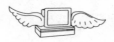

pain has nothing to do with your workstation, but results from your peering forward to see because your eyesight needs correction. A useful solution can be elusive, because it must result from a knowledge and respect for the entire office ecosystem. All aspects of the office must exist in harmony to minimize stress on its most important inhabitant: you.

Dangers of Delay

Like a natural ecosystem, when something goes out of whack in the office, it might not be immediately obvious. Your body and your mind usually compensate, minimizing the immediate effect. People adjust to constrained positions, chairs at the wrong height, and bosses who put them in lousy moods. But when the adjustment becomes chronic, the body becomes ripe for injury. Most computer-related injuries result from the accumulation of repeated stresses and minor injuries. The trick to working safely in the office ecosystem is ensuring that no factor in the environment puts undue stress on your body or your mind. You must be comfortable—physically and mentally—to ensure good health.

Judgment Off the Job

You can't separate the stresses and strains of the job from what you experience off the job. Leisure activities such as golf, tennis, gardening, or playing a musical instrument may have you repeatedly moving body parts in the same way as you do at work, thereby complicating or worsening your injuries. Is it your typing that's hurting you, or pulling dandelions on weekends? Often it's impossible to know with certainty. The entire range of your activities must be viewed together when preventing and treating the repetitive strains and other injuries often associated with computer use.

Prevention and Early Intervention

As the ad says: You can pay me now or pay me later. Often, the longer computer-related injuries are ignored, the more difficult it is to fix them. Letting a bad situation go on for too long can lead to permanent disability. Don't let it happen to you. Prevention and early intervention (both medical treatment and modification of the workplace and job) are the keys to reducing computer-health problems.

Be sure to listen to your body; when something hurts, intervene in a constructive way. If you don't take the time to be healthy now, you may be forced to take the time to be sick later.

BODY & MIND

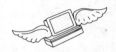

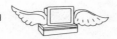

1. The Eyes Have It

Each year 10 million Americans see optometrists for computer-related eye complaints.

■ ■ ■

Most of us take our eyesight for granted—until we overwork or over stress our eyes. Then our eyes may protest in the form of eyestrain—the health complaint most often heard from computer users. Consider these steps to help you watch out for your eyes.

Eyestrain Tip-Offs

- **Focusing problems.** Soft or fuzzy vision is the most common signal of eyestrain.

- **Double vision.** Staring at a close object (like your monitor) can stress your eye-alignment muscles. This can result in a headache or generalized fatigue, and eventually double vision—especially if you already have a marginal problem in keeping your eyes aligned.

- **Headaches.** Most computer-related headaches first begin as tension in the neck and head muscles—a common result of attempting to see in adverse conditions. See page 16.

- **Symptoms on a schedule.** Do the eye problems you have all week disappear over the weekend? Such a recurring pattern is one indication of computer-caused eyestrain.

- **Color confusion.** Many people worry when they look away from their monitors and notice that colors seem bleached out or shifted. Don't worry. This harmless effect disappears within minutes.

Watch Out!

- As many as 40% of people intensively using computers experience eyestrain. Long periods of repeatedly shifting focus, or holding the same focus for too long, can cause eyestrain.

- Poor workstation conditions, such as glare, reflections, bright lights, and dimly lit reading materials can set the stage for eyestrain.

- Avoid having your screen and reading material at extremely different distances. It forces you to repeatedly change focus.

- You may need glasses, or a new prescription, and you may not even know it. Sight sufficient for other tasks often doesn't stand up to the demands of computer work.

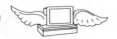

- Glasses themselves can cause problems—bifocal wearers may tilt their heads back, creating eyestrain and perhaps neck and back problems. See page 13.

- A high amount of psychological stress, on and off the job, is associated with eyestrain.

- **Warning.** Some eyestrain symptoms can be caused by a serious condition or disease. Do not hesitate to see an eye-care specialist.

Steps to Take

Pauses that refresh:

- Glance away from your monitor to relax your eye muscles. Dr. Jim Sheedy of U.C. Berkeley's VDT Eye Clinic suggests looking away from the computer every 10 minutes or so and refocusing as far as possible into the distance for five or 10 seconds.

- Try to apportion any work you do off the computer throughout your workday.

- Take breaks away from your workstation to relax both your eyes and your body. Bonus: Rest breaks are known to have a beneficial effect on overall job performance. See page 28.

- Practice stress-reduction techniques during breaks. Find a comfortable position, close your eyes, breathe deeply, and imagine yourself in a peaceful setting.

Peeper protection:

- Get an eye examination once a year, even if you only work on a computer occasionally. See page 12.

- Control the lights and monitor. Try to maintain an even level of lighting around your computer, avoiding any "hot spots" in your field of vision. Ensure that your monitor is adjusted properly and the screen is clean. See pages 46–51.

- Place reading materials on a clip or copy stand adjacent to the monitor. Position the monitor 18" or more from your eyes (if you have good vision), and at a downward gaze angle. See page 49.

Resource

20/20: A Total Guide to Improving Your Vision and Preventing Eye Disease. Mitchell H. Friedlaender and Stef Donvev (Emmaus, Pennsylvania: Rodale Press, 1991). Our favorite easy-to-read handbook about all aspects of eye care.

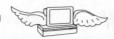

2. Glasses & Contacts

*30% of working-age people in the U.S. have an uncorrected
or inadequately corrected vision problem.*

■ ■ ■

Millions of people have problems seeing the computer monitor, for three
major reasons. First, computer work is particularly demanding on the
eyes—so even if you can see well in other situations, you might not see a
computer screen clearly. Second, many forms of eyesight correction
cause problems at the computer. Third, eyesight worsens as you age, so if
you have no problems now, just wait.

Say, Can You See?

- Generally, computer users stare at the screen for long periods, placing
  stress on the muscles that focus and direct the eye.

- Computer users often make the same eye movements repeatedly,
  fatiguing their eye muscles.

- Many computer screens aren't very bright, which makes the eye work
  harder to focus. This is especially true of monitors that display light
  letters on a dark background.

- Computer users often work in dry environments, and tend not to
  blink often, which decreases the lubricating layer of tears on the eye.

Signals That You May Need Glasses

**The American Optometric Association suggests you should have your
vision checked if you experience:**

- Frequent headaches
- Blurred vision, or tired or burning eyes
- Difficulty parking or frequent accidents
- Difficulty reading the newspaper or other small print
- Poor sports performance
- Decreased interest in tasks requiring close work

WARNING! Seek an immediate eye examination if you experience:

- A profound change in vision
- Eye discomfort for any prolonged period
- Wandering eyes or double vision
- Finding you cover one eye when you read

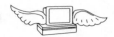

As We Get Older:

- Our eyes' lenses harden, impairing our ability to focus on nearby objects, like computer screens. This natural loss of near vision, called presbyopia, happens to everyone.

- Our pupils become smaller, allowing less light to enter the eye. As a result, we need more light to see well.

- There is a tendency for the eye's lens to yellow, and for cataracts (clouding of the eye's lens) to develop. Cataracts can scatter light— making bright lights or reflections more visually incapacitating.

- Tear production decreases, especially in women. This makes eyes already dried by computer use even more irritated. See page 15.

Hazards of Glasses

Many bifocals, trifocals, and contact lenses that aren't prescribed for use with computers can cause various symptoms.

- **Bifocals and trifocals**. Standard prescriptions work well for reading material on a desk or in your hands, but can cause you to cock your head back and move it forward to clearly see a computer screen—a "chicken dance" that can result in neck and back strain.

- **Contact lenses**. Normal contact lenses are designed to focus at 20 feet so may be inadequate for nearer distances, especially at the low light levels of many monitors. At the computer, contact lens wearers are particularly susceptible to dry eyes.

- **Progressive addition lenses** contain variable-power in one unit: the top part of the lens focuses on objects far away, while the lower parts focus on progressively closer objects. Many wearers find typical progressive addition lenses taxing for long periods at the monitor. However, some newer models are less stressful.

Steps to Take

Adjust your workstation:

- If your bifocals make you cock your head back to see, try lowering your monitor.

- Increase the size of text on your monitor so you don't need vision correction to read it.

- Check to see if your vision problems are due to bright spots or reflections. See page 46.

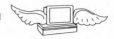

Have an eye examination:

- The AOA suggests you have an eye examination before you begin computer work, and follow-up exams at yearly intervals.

- Increasing numbers of eye-care professionals understand the special factors involved in computer-related eye issues, and will analyze your vision for your work situation. You may receive a prescription for glasses customized for your computing environment.

- **Tip**: Tell the examiner you think you have a computer-related eye problem. If you are asked for a description of the distances and angles from your eyes to your screen, keyboard, and documents, then the examiner probably has the experience you want. Otherwise, consider another examiner.

The Right Correction

About 40% of those who see optometrists about computer-related eye problems receive lenses customized to computer work.

- **Computer glasses** are designed for the distance and angle at which you view your monitor. No one wants to pay for an additional pair of glasses, but many people report that the resulting decrease in eyestrain is well worth the extra cost.

- **Bifocals**. Examiners may prescribe bifocals in which the top lens corrects for objects at monitor distance (with the bottom lens set for closer work). Some people may find relief by lowering their monitors. Sometimes larger bifocals may be prescribed to increase the area of good focus at the monitor's distance.

- **Contacts**. Bifocal contacts can be a satisfactory solution for those who don't want to wear glasses—but they don't work for everyone—and around the computer they have the same drawbacks as other types of contact lenses.

Resources

Both of these organizations will supply free information on computer work and eye health:

American Academy of Ophthalmology. PO Box 7424, San Francisco, CA 94120-7424. (415) 561-8500.

The American Optometric Association. 243 North Lindbergh Blvd., St. Louis, MO 63141. (314) 991- 4100.

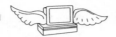

3. Dry Eyes

Computer use can dry your eyes.

■ ■ ■

Go ahead and cry: the eye needs the lubrication of tears to function properly. A lack of lubricating tears makes the eyes scratchy, red, and irritated. Even if you've never looked at a computer, factors like your age and what medications you take can reduce your production of tears. But what most people don't realize is that particular aspects of computer use can dry eyes, too.

How Dry Am Eyes?

■ People blink considerably less often when using computers, so tears don't spread over the eye's surface as they should.

■ If you stare at an object high in your visual field—where most people's monitors are located—you open the eyelids more, resulting in increased tear evaporation.

■ As you get older, your tear production decreases; this is especially true in women—it's not known why.

■ The air circulation systems in office buildings typically dry the air, as can the heat generated by your computer.

■ Many medications, such as diuretics and antihistamines, can reduce the production of lubricating tears.

Steps to Take

■ **Think to blink**. Whether or not you use eye drops, blink often—at least every five seconds—to keep eyes properly lubricated.

■ **Lower your monitor** to expose less of the eye's surface and reduce tear evaporation. But make sure your monitor still is at a comfortable viewing height.

■ **Moisten the air**. Home workers can use a humidifier or set out bowls of water to put some H_2O in the air. In an office building, tell your manager if you believe that the air is too dry.

■ **Use eye drops**. Over-the-counter eye drops are a quick remedy for dry eyes. Eye experts suggest that if you use eye drops, get those that are just lubricants, based on methyl cellulose or polyvinyl alcohol. Eye drops containing decongestants or vasoconstrictors can result in a rebound effect, actually causing the eye to dry.

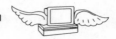

4. Have I Got a Headache!

Headaches come in many varieties.

■ ■ ■

Do computers cause headaches? No, except perhaps in extremely rare circumstances. But many of the things that trigger headaches—deadlines, heavy work loads, repetitive and monotonous tasks, air quality, and glaring lights—are common in computer workplaces.

Headaches are hard for science to pin down; they appear in different sizes, shapes, and varieties. Their origins defy neat classification because they develop from interrelating functions of the brain, neck, and head. But luckily for us, science has had success in treatment.

Guide to the Headache Galaxy

- **Tension headaches,** the most common of headache types, are linked to a tensing, or contracting, of the head and neck muscles, causing pain. Bad posture at your workstation and poor workstation setup are prime causes of tension.

- **Migraine headaches.** Usually attacking one side of the head, migraines are linked to disturbances in the blood vessels serving the head and brain, and seem to be hereditary. Migraines are often triggered by external stimuli: light, noises, certain foods, stress, pain, the menstrual cycle, and even smells, like paint fumes.

- **Less common headaches.** Ice cream, coughing, depression, sinus problems, and even sex can cause headaches. Sometimes headaches can be caused by an underlying illness or condition, such as a tumor, infection, or disease.

Steps to Prevention

- **Be aware.** Pay attention to the intensity and frequency of headaches. Some migraine and chronic tension headache sufferers can determine what prompts an episode and then try to avoid the triggers.

- **Limit stress.** Maintaining a relaxed and comfortable work environment is one of the most effective ways of preventing tension headaches. See page 32.

- **Reduce muscle strains and pulls** by practicing good posture at a workstation that adequately supports the upper body, neck, and shoulders. Consider a telephone headset; a standard handset causes strain when crooked against your neck. See page 20.

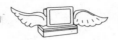

- **Optimize your view of the screen.** Make sure the monitor is directly in front of you at an appropriate distance and height. Eliminate reflections in the monitor. Consider an antiglare screen. Experiment with screen brightness and contrast. See page 48.

- **Focus on fresh air.** If you smell something funny, such as paint or solvent vapors, report it; some chemical vapors can cause headaches and more serious health problems. Note if you became aware of any new odors around the same time you started getting headaches.

- **Watch what you eat.** Certain foods trigger headaches in some people. Pay attention to intake of sulfides, present in many red wines; monosodium glutamate (MSG), found in Chinese and many prepared foods; and nitrites, often found in meats, and in aged and processed cheeses.

Treatment

- Don't be a martyr: headaches can indicate serious ailments. If your headaches bother you, see a doctor.

- Migraine sufferers should be under the care of a doctor; most find relief with prescription medications.

- If you get a headache every time you look at your monitor, see your doctor—you may be one of the rare people who some specialists suggest may have headaches triggered by computer screens. Glare shields, dark glasses, adjusting screen color and brightness, or an LCD screen may help.

- For an occasional tension headache, over-the-counter pain relievers—aspirin, ibuprofen, or acetaminophen—may do the trick. But dependence on pain relievers can backfire, causing more headaches. If headaches persist, see a doctor. See page 65.

- Either cold or hot compresses can ease a variety of headaches. But migraine sufferers beware: applying heat can often worsen migraines.

- Relaxation techniques—such as biofeedback, meditation, and relaxation exercises—may help.

Resources

National Headache Foundation. 5252 North Western Avenue, Chicago, Illinois 60625. (312) 878-7715. They will provide information on headaches and treatment.

Most cities and major hospitals have headache clinics; consult your Yellow Pages under **Hospitals**.

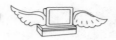

5. Watch Your Back

Back problems can creep up, worsening with time.

■ ■ ■

Just sitting stresses the back and neck; the longer you sit, the more the strain. Sitting tends to tilt the pelvis backward, flattening the lumbar curve (the inward bend at the small of the back), which can result in uneven and increased pressure on spinal disks.

Back Facts

- 80% of people experience lower back pain at some time. Fortunately, most back pain resolves itself.

- Up to 85% of back pain cannot be diagnosed definitively.

- Diagnosis is difficult because back injuries can be felt elsewhere in the body. Pain or tingling in the foot, for example, may mean nerve damage in the spine.

Where Does It Hurt?

- Generalized back and neck pain can be due to muscle fatigue. Sitting statically or forcing muscles into tensed positions for long hours reduces blood circulation, so lactic acid—a product of muscle action that's usually flushed away by the blood—can build up, producing aches and sores.

- Lower back pain may be produced by a variety of posture problems including slouching, leaning forward, or sitting with your feet dangling.

- Pain in the upper back and neck can result from slouching, improper upper back support, or working in a twisted position.

- Irritation of the spine or compression of nerves or veins can result from sitting for long periods, especially on hard seats with protruding surfaces.

- Double-crush syndrome occurs when a nerve is pinched in two places: at the neck (or a little below) and at the hands or wrists. The two nerve pinches combined may result in numbness, tingling, or weakness in the hands, arms, shoulder, or upper back.

- Stiffness, muscle spasm, and radiating pain in the neck or upper back may be caused by chronic neck-muscle strain known as tension neck syndrome. Constantly staring at a screen for long periods strains the neck muscles that keep the head balanced over the spine.

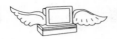

- Numbness, tingling, and pain in the back or the neck may be the result of serious afflictions, such as herniated disks, tumors, or degenerative diseases.

Steps to Take

A few simple steps may help prevent or relieve back problems.

- Sit sensibly. See page 20.
- Mild or occasional back pain may be relieved by using over-the-counter pain medicines such as aspirin or ibuprofen.

See a doctor if you experience:

- Persistent pain, numbness, or tingling
- Acute or chronic pain
- Any changes in urination or bowel function

Practice back safety everywhere.

- Squat to pick up heavy loads and use leg muscles when lifting.
- Exercise regularly to improve blood circulation and strengthen the muscles that help support the spine.
- Walking is an excellent exercise for the back, easy on the spine.
- Listen to your mother: don't slouch, stand with shoulders back, head high, letting your back curve naturally, tilt your pelvis forward, stomach tucked in, and don't lock your knees.
- If prolonged standing is necessary, put one foot on a stool or thick phone book. Periodically alternate the supporting foot.

Good News in Diagnosis and Treatment

- MRI and CAT scans, both relatively recent advances, can image soft tissue, including nerves, giving doctors a better view of possible problems in the back than is available with X-ray techniques.
- For those requiring back surgery, new, less invasive procedures may be helpful. If you need back surgery, ask your doctor about new arthroscopic techniques (where instruments are inserted through small incisions) which may decrease both complications and recovery time.

Resources

Texas Back Institute. (800) 247-BACK. Will answer questions and provide material about back problems.

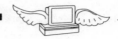

6. Sit Sensibly

Every moment you sit upright, hundreds of muscles are hard at work, fighting gravity.

■ ■ ■

Sitting is a compromise. You sit to reduce the strain on your muscles, allowing them a chance to rest and recuperate. But, simultaneously, other muscles work to keep you sitting.

Facts to Sit On

- Humans are not designed to sit. Even if your posture is perfect, the pressure on the lumbar disks (the doughnut-shaped cartilage between the vertebrae in your spine) increases by 30% when you are seated.

- Studies by NASA in zero gravity demonstrated that a relaxed body configured itself somewhere between sitting and lying down.

- Experts are still learning what's the best seated posture, and exactly how comfort relates to injury levels.

Start by Adjusting Your Workstation

- Make sure the computer screen sits directly in front of you; keep reading material within comfortable sight, at eye level or below; and keep telephones within easy reach.

- Adjust your chair so your body feels relaxed and comfortable, with nothing pressing into it. If you don't know how to adjust your chair, find out.

- If your chair's lumbar support is insufficient, you might be able to use a cushion or "roll" to provide this support. Make sure the support doesn't push you into an awkward posture.

- For a typical upright position, adjust your chair height so you can hang your arms straight down from your shoulders with your elbows bent 90 degrees to allow you to comfortably place your fingers on your keyboard with your wrists in a neutral position. Your feet should be flat on the floor or a footrest.

Next Step: Sit Right

- When sitting upright, keep your feet flat on the floor or a footrest.
- Don't slump your shoulders. Keep your chin slightly tucked in.

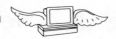

- Maintain your lumbar curve. The back of your chair should support your lower back, so use it—don't sit forward and lean over. Placing a rolled-up towel or pillow in the small of your back may help.
- Avoid twisting, jerking, or repetitively bending the neck.
- Don't hold a telephone between your shoulder and cheek.
- Keep fidgeting; even small changes in position help avoid overtaxing certain muscles or parts of the spine.

Take the Posture Test

- Are you unsure whether you are sitting correctly? Good posture is usually evident to the eye, so have a co-worker check out your posture at your workstation. Work alone at home? Pull your chair over to a full-length mirror and check yourself out.

Re: Position

- Determine two working positions that are comfortable yet different. Then switch between them regularly. Reclining is easiest on the back, but make sure your neck is supported. Detachable keyboards can help you recline.
- If possible, alternate between sitting and standing. Many workplaces are accepting standing as a viable computing posture.

Take Active Breaks

- At break time, don't stay in your chair. Take pressure off the spine and get the blood pumping by moving around. Walk around the office, jump up and down, go outside for fresh air.
- Sometimes your body may be telling you to put your feet up. Go ahead. Although this may seem to be an "unprofessional" posture, stretching out for short periods reduces pressure on your discs and allows fatigued muscles to relax and recuperate. Don't try working at the keyboard while stretching out—just relax!

References

Sitting on the Job: How to Survive the Stresses of Sitting Down to Work. Scott Donkin (Boston: Houghton Mifflin Company, 1989). A chiropractor looks at sitting from all the angles.

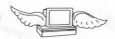

7. A Healthy Hand

Cumulative trauma disorders are the fastest growing workers' compensation claim.

■ ■ ■

A twinge of hand pain makes many of us fear we have carpal tunnel syndrome. Possible, but unlikely. Carpal tunnel syndrome has gotten a lot of press—but it's less common than many other injuries associated with computer use. Injuries due to repetitive movement, like those made at a computer, are called cumulative trauma disorders (CTDs). CTDs occur when a body part repeatedly receives small traumas—eventually accumulating a wear that can be painful and disabling.

CTD Facts

- CTDs are often subtle affairs, developing slowly over time. Even those who type lightly and infrequently can eventually develop CTDs.

- With CTDs, it's common for several injuries to occur at once, causing multiple symptoms that may be tricky to pinpoint. Weakness in one body part affects related body parts. Tingling in the hand, for example, could be related to a problem in the forearm.

Will You Develop a CTD?

It is impossible to say who will develop a cumulative trauma disorder. But watch out for these factors associated with CTD development:

- Awkward postures put uneven stress on body parts, leading to myriad problems, particularly of the back and wrists.

- Constantly flexing the hands up and down by bending the wrists is believed to be a major contributor to carpal tunnel syndrome.

- Typing with twisted or cocked wrists or forearms not parallel to the floor can cause strain. Letting your wrists or forearms rest on a surface while you type may overwork and stress the muscles in your hands. Pounding the keys puts stress on the fingers.

- Demands of the job like deadlines or long periods of repetitive typing are associated with CTDs.

- Working at cold temperatures may increase the chance of developing CTDs. Poor diet, lack of sleep, and smoking can all be risks.

- Your body's particular physiology may predispose you to certain CTDs, and diseases like alcoholism and diabetes are also seen to be contributing factors.

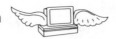

Warning Signs of CTDs

Note: CTDs can cause a variety of symptoms, and early symptoms can be hard to notice, so many computer users may not realize that problems are underway. When any of the following symptoms occurs (especially if it persists or becomes chronic), see a medical professional:

- Burning pain during noncomputer time, particularly during your normal sleeping hours
- Localized pain or dull achiness, with or without movement
- Radiating pain that travels up and down the arm or shoulder
- Numbness, tingling, weakness, or stiffness
- Loss of muscle coordination or control

Steps to Recovery

- Start by admitting you have a problem. Feeling that you can overcome or ride out symptoms on your own can be dangerous. Long-term problems can cause permanent and painful disability.
- Let a medical professional, preferably with a background in CTDs, guide your treatment. Doctors can employ a variety of specialized tests to aid accurate diagnoses of CTDs. Specific problems usually require specific treatments, making medical diagnosis critical.
- Occasional or mild CTD symptoms may disappear with rest and the use of over-the-counter anti-inflammatory pain relievers (such as aspirin or ibuprofen).
- Many people find relief by icing or using alternating hot and cold water baths. But when experiencing acute or recurring symptoms, self-treatment isn't advised—see a health professional.
- Arm or wrist splints and slings, arm rests, wrist rests, and other apparatus advertised as preventing or treating CTDs can further damage an existing problem if they aren't used properly.
- Medical treatments include simple rest, anti-inflammatory medications or injections, physical therapy, or—in extreme cases—surgery.

Preventative Steps

Work defensively.

- Create diversity in your work tasks to avoid long periods of time in the same movement. Take frequent short rest breaks from repetitive keystroking. See page 28.
- Try warm-up or break exercises and stretches. Stay warm. See page 25.

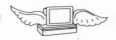

- Watch out for pushing or resting wrists or forearms against hard desk edges. See page 20.
- Adjust your workstation; position your keyboard. See page 20.

Straighten those wrists.

- Keep the hands flat and even with the wrists and forearms. This is best achieved through proper positioning of the desk and keyboard. Avoid constantly stretching the hands side to side.

Be mindful of mouse movements.

- Try to avoid overstretching the fingers or thumbs. Don't extend your pinkies. Keep the mouse in easy reach from the keyboard, and be gentle; don't grab or tap the mouse forcefully. See page 44.

Pay attention to posture.

- Bad posture often develops in childhood or over long periods of time and can be very difficult to correct. Try to maintain a periodic awareness of your body throughout the day.

- Sit in a comfortable position that evenly distributes weight over your spine, while supporting your lumbar curve. Arms should extend comfortably from the elbow so that hands can use the keyboard without bending up or down at the wrist. Don't slouch forward or round your shoulders.

- Avoid developing dangerous habits such as pressing the forearms into the desk edge, tilting the head towards the window, planting one arm on an arm rest, and so forth. Change positions frequently.

Play smart.

- Injuries suffered off the job often worsen on the job. It's a cycle with no clear starting point. Any activity that involves force, repetition, and postural changes can put you at risk for CTDs. Listen to your body while at play, and stop when it tells you to.

Resources

The Carpal Tunnel Syndrome Book. Mark A. Pinsky (New York: Warner Books, 1993). An inexpensive paperback that provides comprehensive information on CTDs.

Repetitive Strain Injury: A Computer User's Guide. Emil Pascarelli and Deborah Quilter (New York: John Wiley and Sons, Inc., 1994).

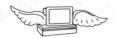

8. Move It!

Sitting too long can injure you.

■ ■ ■

The trend at many companies in recent years has been to reduce mobility of the worker—put the computer user in a chair for the entire day, every day. That's wrong. The human body is not designed for sitting for long periods.

To perform well, the body needs to regularly move through its natural range of motion—keeping joints lubricated and muscles toned. Movement is good for you, and with a little effort your workday can become part of an overall fitness program.

Priority One: Move!

- If you could only do one thing to make yourself safer at the computer it should be: move.
- Shifting position in your chair rotates stress between different muscle groups, allowing some muscles to rest and recuperate, while other muscles work.
- Getting up and walking down the hall relaxes your hands, wrists, arms, back, neck, eyes, and mind.
- Taking breaks increases productivity. Get up and go.

Before You Exercise

Exercise can be very beneficial, but it isn't for every body.

- **Think.** Start slowly. Not doing any exercise is safer than overdoing it when you are out of shape. Listen to your body; never stretch to the point of pain or discomfort. Use your common sense.
- **Think twice.** Stretches or exercise can worsen some cumulative trauma disorders, even incipient problems you are unaware of. To be safe, check with a doctor to ensure that stretching or exercise is right for you—especially if you've had recent surgery or haven't exercised regularly for some time.
- **And note.** Breaks without exercise help, too: a National Institute of Occupational Safety and Health office study showed that passive breaks improved mood and comfort just as much as breaks incorporating exercise.

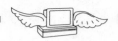

Integrate Exercise into Your Workday

- **Use the stairs.** Stairs are a great way to improve cardiovascular performance and stamina.

- **Park about a five-minute walk away from the office.** Or, if you live less than a few miles from work, consider walking. Brisk walking is a great way to start your day and loosen up on the way home.

- **Run errands at lunch.** Maybe not run, but walk quickly. See how much you can accomplish in a limited period, but don't get stressed!

- **Use leisure activities** to exercise your neglected muscles, instead of straining those that are overworked. Swimming and jogging are generally good alternatives for a computer user.

Warm Up Before Work and Throughout the Day

Posture Stretch

- Sit straight, maintaining a lumbar curve.
- Reach both arms straight up, as high as you can, while imagining a rope pulling your head straight up.
- Allow arms to slowly drop into your lap, and relax your neck.
- Repeat five times.

Back Stretch

- Stand straight, and clasp your hands together, placing them in the small of your back.
- Push your hips and hands forward, arching your body.
- Immediately come back to the upright position.
- Repeat five times.

Arms and Shoulders

- Sit straight, slowly raise arms until they are parallel with the floor.
- Slowly rotate arms in small circles.
- Repeat with slow circles in the opposite direction.

Legs and Ankles

- Stretch one leg out and up.
- Move foot around in two complete circles.
- Repeat in other direction.
- Repeat with other foot.

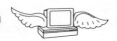

Neck

- Sit straight, eyes looking straight ahead.
- Pull head back, creating a double chin.
- Hold for a few seconds.

Exercise at Your Desk

Each stretch can be performed in sets of up to five repetitions, depending on comfort and time.

Finger Stretch

- Hold your arms straight out in front of you, palms down.
- Spread the fingers apart until you feel resistance.
- Hold for five seconds, then relax.
- Repeat five times.

Hands and Wrists

- Hold left hand in front of you with palm facing up.
- Place palm of right hand onto the fingers of left.
- Using your right hand to provide resistance, try to press the fingers of left hand up.
- Switch hand positions and repeat.

Look Away

- Every 10 minutes look away from the screen and focus on the most distant object available for 10 seconds. This should be done just once, not in repetition.

References

Stretch and Strengthen. Judy Alter (Boston: Houghton Mifflin, 1986). Our favorite book on stretching.

Stretching. Bob Anderson (New York: Random House, 1980). An encyclopedia of stretches, and how to do them.

"A review of physical exercises recommended for VDT operators." *Applied Ergonomics*, Vol. 23, No. 6, December 1992. This NIOSH review of the usefulness and safety of 127 office exercises is dense but interesting reading. Most of the exercises were found to be potentially stressful and could possibly lead to injury.

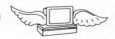

9. Right on Schedule

*Most people don't break often
enough or long enough.*

■ ■ ■

The traditional schedule of morning and afternoon work periods, each divided with a 15-minute break, is outdated. While those traditional breaks may serve useful purposes—going to the bathroom, socializing, getting a snack—they aren't frequent enough to allow the body to recover from the stress related to computer work. A schedule with more frequent but shorter breaks increases productivity and comfort, but there is no exact formula for the perfect work/rest schedule.

Break for Efficiency

A recent NIOSH study tested a schedule of three-minute breaks every 40 to 50 minutes, with 30-second micropauses every 10 minutes. During their breaks, users were told to do something other than work at their computers.

■ The results of the study showed a decrease in worker discomfort—and a significant increase in productivity—compared to the traditional schedule of midmorning and midafternoon breaks.

■ Two insurance companies that instituted this schedule found the efficiency of claims processing was higher during the test period than in a typical earlier period.

Breaking Down the Break

Dr. Robert A. Henning, a psychology professor in industrial organization at the University of Connecticut, says that computer users "don't break early enough, often enough, or long enough." All break schedules should meet the following criteria:

■ Breaks need to be taken in advance of pain. If you break after you begin to feel discomfort, it will take much longer to recover than if you take a break earlier.

■ Breaks need to be long enough to allow recovery. Spontaneous breaks are often only five to 10 seconds—not sufficient to allow for recovery from strain.

■ Breaks need to be taken often enough. Muscle stress recovery needs to go on throughout the working day to maintain low stress levels.

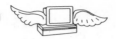

Steps Away from Your Work

While authorities differ as to how often and how long computer users should pause for breaks, most have upped the recommended numbers over the past several years.

- The Occupational Medicine Clinic at San Francisco General Hospital recommends a 10-minute break (or alternate work) at least once an hour, and a computing day of four to six hours.

- US West and AT&T reduced CTD symptoms by providing one-minute "mini-breaks" every 20 minutes.

- NIOSH has recommended a 15-minute break for every two hours of moderately demanding VDT work (or for every one hour of intensive VDT use).

- The NIOSH study discussed earlier suggests that the schedule of a three-minute break every 50 minutes with 30-second breaks every 10 minutes is also effective.

- In his book, *Repetitive Strain Injury: A Computer User's Guide,* hand expert Dr. Emil Pascarelli suggests, "If you are not injured, take a 5- to 10-minute break from typing for every half hour that you work. One break per hour should include stretching: the other should be spent doing nonkeyboard activities."

Resources

9to5, National Association of Working Women. 238 West Wisconsin Ave., Suite 700, Milwaukee, WI 53203-2308. (414) 274-0925. 9to5 is a membership organization run mostly by volunteers in local chapters. 9to5 focuses on protecting the rights of office workers. They have a job problem hotline—(800) 522-0925—for people to call who are experiencing or witnessing work-related problems of any kind.

National Institute of Occupational Safety and Health (NIOSH). Technical Information Branch, Mail Stop C19, 4676 Columbia Parkway, Cincinnati, OH 45226. Information line: (800) 356-4674. NIOSH will provide information about seeking local assistance in occupational health issues, but they do not refer people directly to other agencies or services.

Labor Occupational Health Program. School of Public Health, University of California at Berkeley, 2515 Channing Way, 2nd Floor, Berkeley, CA 94720. (510) 642-5507. Nonprofit organization that provides job safety and health information, mainly to workers and the public. Maintains library and publishes educational material.

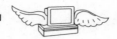

10. An Apple a Day

Lack of good health makes a computer user more vulnerable to muscle strains, aches, and pains.

■ ■ ■

You've been told over and over to pay attention to your diet, get enough sleep, exercise regularly, avoid harmful substances, and so forth. But if you really want to be safer at your workstation, you need to take good health—the foundation of safe computing—seriously.

Unsafer Computing

- Computer use can be hard work, employing thousands of back, neck, torso, arm, and leg muscles. Out-of-shape muscles are more prone to stress, strain, and pain.

- Chronic sleep disorders are extremely common. Lack of sleep lowers performance and mood, and makes one more prone to injury.

- Most computer work involves psychological stress, and chronic stress is linked to computer injury as well as a variety of mental and physical health problems.

- Improper diet can promote illness, injury, and low moods.

- Cigarette smoking, or alcohol or drug abuse are linked to long-term health problems and can affect one's mental well being—even if one abstains in the office.

Steps to Take

Get regular exercise.

- Regular exercise improves cardiovascular fitness and builds muscle strength, which increases muscle efficiency and helps prevent strain.

- Specialists recommend heart-pumping exercise at least three times a week, for at least 20 minutes.

- If it's been awhile since you've made your body work, get your doctor's advice on how to ease into an exercise regime slowly.

Get a good night's sleep.

If you can't fall asleep, or wake up and can't get back to sleep:

- Try getting out of bed, going to a different room, and finding a relaxing activity: reading, working a crossword puzzle, writing, or taking a bath. Then, when you start to feel drowsy, go back to bed.

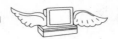

- Try avoiding caffeine later in the day. Try ear plugs or a sleep mask to block noise and light. For occasional insomnia, over-the-counter medicines may help, but don't make them a habit.

- Don't drink alcohol to try to make yourself sleepy. Most alcohol has sugar which can wake you up after it enters your blood stream.

- Consult a doctor if sleep difficulties persist.

Take time to relax.

- Make deep relaxation a priority off the job. Give yourself down time to make up for the hours of on time demanded at work.

- Regular exercise, massage, and meditation are proven relaxants; you probably have your own. Incorporate as many of them into your regular routine as possible.

Eat properly.

- Eat a balanced diet that's low in fat and high in fruits, vegetables, and grains.

- Start each day with a solid breakfast and don't skip meals, which can lead to stomach pains and lethargy.

- Snack wisely. Fruits and vegetables and popcorn (without butter) are healthy low-calorie snacks. Sugar is used up quickly and supplies almost no nutrients.

- If you're trying to lose or gain weight, consult a doctor first. Many diets aren't nutritionally balanced and will affect your daily energy level and mood.

- Drink plenty of fluids, but don't rely on the caffeine found in coffee, tea, and many soft drinks to charge your day. Caffeine enhances alertness, but too much caffeine can backfire, leading to a dependence that's associated with mood swings and headaches.

Check in now and then.

- Blood pressure, cholesterol levels, and weight are a few things that can help gauge health. Have these checked periodically—every couple of years, or more often if you have a known concern.

Seek help for habits.

- Many larger businesses offer confidential employee assistance programs to help break addictions. For people who must seek help from an outside source, many organizations, hospitals, and clinics provide excellent services.

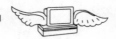

11. Not to Worry

*Costs to industry from job stress
exceed $150 billion a year.*

■ ■ ■

High amounts of psychological stress are linked to various forms of
computer injury. Is it a wonder? Most computer work teems with stress
sources: from monotonous keyboarding to lack of social interaction to
static postures. Because everyone reacts differently to stress, a stress level
appropriate for you may be inappropriate for a co-worker. The trick is
finding a balance between positive, motivating stress and stress overload.

Did You Know?

■ Chronic stress may be linked to a whole range of health problems—
some serious—including heart disease, high cholesterol, hypertension,
ulcers, exhaustion, anxiety, and depression.

■ Less serious but potentially debilitating conditions linked to stress
include head-, back-, and neckaches; insomnia; upper respiratory
infections; and skin rashes such as psoriasis and eczema.

■ For most people, a little stress, off and on, is a positive, energizing
stimulant. Boredom can be a damaging stressor.

■ A 1990 study by Johns Hopkins University found that the occupations
with the highest number of workers suffering from depression
included secretaries, typists, data entry keyboarders, and computer
equipment operators.

Your Body's Steps to Stress Overload

1. Demands from the outside world are perceived as threats or calls
to action.

2. In response, the adrenal glands pump out two hormones, cortisol
and adrenaline, that raise heart rates, blood pressure, and blood flow.

3. Simultaneously, blood sugar is diverted from internal organs to the
brain to increase alertness.

4. After the danger passes, the brain triggers the release of a variety of
substances (including endorphins) that bring the body back to a more
relaxed state.

5. Chronic stress occurs when cortisol and adrenaline levels stay high,
keeping the body in a state of constant alert.

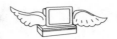

Stress Overload Warnings

Seek medical attention if you experience any of the following symptoms frequently, or their frequency or intensity suddenly increases:

- Frequent headaches
- Frequent backaches, neckaches, or other aches
- Recurring heartburn or acid indigestion
- Bursts of rapid heartbeat
- Sleep disturbances
- Increased bad moods or anger
- Constant tension; feeling wound up or on edge
- Unusual lethargy, exhaustion, or apathy
- Hives or skin rashes
- Increased drug or alcohol use

Steps to Reduce Stress

Bear in mind the three Rs: relaxation, reduction, and reorientation. Stress management should be a combination of reducing exposure to stressors, relaxing—quieting the stressed-out body, and reorienting expectations and self-demands.

Plan ahead.

- Schedule to meet deadlines. Use planning to avoid stressful work back-ups and overloads. Take as much control in your work schedule as the job allows.

Fight monotony.

- If you are feeling bored and restless, look for ways to make your work more challenging. Most of us fear change, but mastering new challenges can be invigorating.
- Ask for more responsibility, ask to learn new technology, brainstorm new ideas with co-workers, consider switching to another department.

Consider alternatives.

- Breaking routine can often reduce stress. Some companies offer methods to personalize or tailor the work schedule, such as flex time and job sharing.
- Some companies allow for leaves of absence to take classes or to do volunteer work or community service.

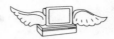

Exercise during the workday.

■ Park your car in the far corner of the parking lot. Take the stairs instead of the elevator. Get up and walk to someone's desk instead of relying on e-mail.

■ Break for several minutes each hour and wiggle your fingers, take your eyes off the screen, stand up and stretch, walk around your office, practice relaxation.

■ On larger breaks, find a place in the office to exercise, chat with co-workers, get fresh air, find a quiet place to shut your eyes, or jog around the block. Everyone's different, so tap into the force that lifts your spirits.

Eat well.

■ Start with a healthy breakfast.

■ Eat carbohydrates for long-lasting energy. Light, nutritious lunches and frequent healthy snacks—nuts, fruit, crackers—are better energizers than large meals eaten less frequently.

■ Drink plenty of fluids throughout the day, but watch for dependence on caffeine or sugary soft drinks; they may be linked to moodiness or depression.

Talk it out.

■ Get work frustrations off your chest by talking about them with family and friends. Talking can be an excellent way to release bottled-up feelings, but avoid falling into a mode of constant complaining.

■ Many larger businesses have counselors on staff who are experts in job stress. Consider seeking their help.

Take action.

■ If job stress becomes a major concern, it may be time to discuss problems with a higher authority.

■ Take note of sources of stress that may be affecting large numbers of employees. Approach your supervisor, union representative, or a manager you're comfortable with.

■ Try to stay calm, prepared to negotiate, with positive ideas and suggestions for change.

THE
OFFICE

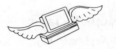

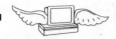

12. A Safer Workstation

*The right equipment, adjusted correctly, provides one
of the cornerstones of safer computing.*

■ ■ ■

Your workstation should be designed and adjusted for your body and
job to minimize physical stress, force, and repetition. But no workstation
can be guaranteed to be injury-free. Training, job design, schedules, and
supervisory relationships need to be considered along with equipment in
producing a healthy computing environment. Adapt this chapter's
contents to your situation.

Steps to Take

- **Keyboard height.** Your elbows should be bent approximately 90° and
  your wrists should be in a flat, "neutral" position. See page 42.

- **Chair.** Your chair should be well-made, and should adjust easily. The
  height should keep your feet comfortably on the floor or a footrest,
  and allow the elbows to bend around 90° while your hands are flat on
  the keyboard. See page 38.

- **Footrest.** You need a footrest if the chair height that's proper for your
  desk doesn't let your feet rest flat on the floor.

- **Bright lights.** Keep bright lights out of your field of vision. Orient
  your workstation to exclude light sources that can't be modified. See
  page 46.

- **Major light sources.** Indirect lighting is preferred; it shouldn't
  overpower the brightness of the screen. See page 46.

- **Task lighting.** Use task lighting only if necessary. Make sure it's not
  too bright and doesn't spill light into your eyes.

- **Reflections.** Control screen reflections by louvering or masking lights,
  repositioning the screen slightly, or attaching a glare shield. See page 46.

- **Room surfaces.** Use matte finishes and neutral tones to reduce
  brightness. See page 46.

- **Noise.** Music and office noise should not be loud enough to annoy or
  distract.

- **Work surface.** Make necessary materials easily accessible. Avoid
  clutter. See page 40.

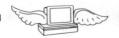

- **Air.** Maintain a comfortable temperature, with adequate fresh air.

- **Space.** You should have enough space to adopt various comfortable positions. Your space should provide some privacy while allowing you to easily shift your focus to a distant object.

- **Monitor.** Ensure adequate resolution, keep it well maintained, and clean the surface regularly. See page 48.

- **Monitor position.** Traditional practice has been that the top of the screen should be at eye height or slightly below, but some experts now say a more downward gaze angle may be better. The monitor should sit at least 18 inches (45 cm) from the eyes, directly in line with the keyboard. See page 48.

- **Electromagnetic fields.** If you are concerned about electromagnetic fields, place the monitor 30 inches (75 cm) away from you unless it meets MPRII (or stricter) standards and stay at least four feet away from the backs or sides of adjacent monitors. See page 54.

- **Type size.** The type displayed on your screen should neither be so small that it's hard to see, nor so large that it slows down your reading. See page 48.

- **Keyboard.** The keyboard should be slim, detached, and provide solid key-press feedback. See page 42.

- **Documents.** If you refer to them often, keep documents on a copy stand adjacent to the screen.

Step Lively

- Shift your seated position frequently to remain comfortable. Adjust your chair and workstation to accommodate.

- Take breaks and alternate tasks. Make it a habit to get up and move away from your workstation.

Step Back

- You need sufficient training (and inclination) to adhere to safety principles. Talk to your supervisor about problems and see your health-care provider if they persist.

- Take proper breaks and consider stretching.

- Keep a positive attitude: lack of job satisfaction makes a worker more prone to suffer the deleterious effects of on-the-job stress.

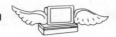

13. The Good Chair

*In one office, researchers found that only 5% of the
adjustable furniture had ever been adjusted.*

■ ■ ■

A good chair is comfortable, adjustable, and adaptable: it maximizes
support and minimizes stress while encouraging you to assume different
positions without "hot spots"—areas where the chair presses on parts of
the body, causing discomfort. The best design accommodates your
workstation, tasks, body, and work intensity.

Common Chair Snares

Back injuries and other problems can be produced by:

- A chair that's too high, which causes you to sit on the front of the seat.
  This position is especially onerous if your feet aren't supported and
  can also lead to sleeping feet and pain under the thigh.

- A chair that's too high *or too low,* which causes you to bend forward.
  Wrist and arm ache can also result because improper chair height
  places your hands and wrists in stressful positions.

- A chair that's neither sufficiently curved nor adequately adjusted to
  hold your lower back in the proper position, causing you to slouch.

- A chair that's positioned too far from your monitor, causing you to
  lean forward to see.

- A chair with a seat that's tilted too far backward, so that your knees are
  drawn up toward your stomach, causing the lumbar curve to flatten.

- A chair with a seat that's poorly contoured or too hard, so that it
  presses into your tailbone or the underside of the thigh.

Chair Notes

- Intensive computer users should have a well-designed chair; those
  whose jobs have them up and down constantly might not require as
  sophisticated a model.

- A well-made chair can appear expensive—until you consider the value
  of its occupant's work, especially in light of medical and disability
  costs. A well-made chair should also last for 20 years (so it should see
  you through many computers at today's turnover rates).

- Not all chairs—even those that appear to be on the forefront of
  design—are based on modern ergonomic principles. Chairs that carry

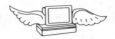

the tag "ergonomic" may or may not be; there is no organization that certifies this elusive quality.

- Chairs should be purchased with a tryout period. If the chair isn't satisfactory, return it.

Steps to Take

Adjust your chair.

- Studies have shown that workers often don't know how to adjust their chairs, and those that do rarely adjust them. Be different; see page 20.

Ponder the perfect chair:

- Chairs are like shoes: you need one in "your size," that provides the right height and support for your body. People who are heavy, short, tall, or thin are all likely to need different chairs.

- The lumbar support, the lower area of the backrest, should adjust vertically to maintain your spine in the correct curvature. If you use a computer for long, intense periods, consider a chair in which you can adjust the contour of the lumbar support.

- The backrest should adjust forward and back to let you adopt at least two comfortable working positions; ideally, it will tilt back as much as 30 degrees to allow you to sit back in a relaxed position. The backrest should extend high enough to provide support when you lean back. A tension adjustment is necessary.

- The seat pan should be padded and contoured for support while allowing movement, and should not touch the leg below your knee. The front should slope down and the surface should provide enough friction to keep you from sliding—but not so much to prevent you from easily shifting position. The pan should tilt forward to give you a range of comfortable working positions.

- Armrests need to be padded and close enough to lean on without straining. They should adjust vertically and not hit or scrape on your workstation.

- A foundation of five legs reduces the chance of accidentally tipping, and casters increase movement. The chair should feel solid. Most people prefer a chair that swivels, but you may not.

- The chair should easily adjust (ideally, while you're sitting in it) to encourage you to change your position. People will more likely adjust the height of chairs that have pneumatic height adjustments.

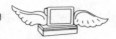

14. Tabling Your Motion

Your desk should function like a cockpit.

■ ■ ■

If you're like most of us, you don't give your desk a second's thought. That's the problem. Most of us accept an ill-conceived, cluttered, and disorganized work space as a fact of life (or a badge of our hard work). Yet how your desk operates—which includes the desk's design and how you work on it—can be critical to your safety.

Ideally, a desk should function like a cockpit—perfectly adapted to fit you and your tasks. The first step is the height of your keyboard, but you also need to consider leg room, workspace, and clutter. A few minutes spent adjusting and organizing your desk can produce significant results.

Common Desk Dangers

- A desk of the wrong height forces you into uncomfortable working postures, stressing your body, especially the wrists and arms.

- A desk without enough leg room prevents you from moving your legs and feet when you work.

- A desk that interferes with chair movement forces you to twist to perform your tasks.

- A desk that doesn't suit your work can stress your body (and your mind). Most common pitfall: the space around the keyboard is too cramped to hold your documents or other necessary materials.

- A desk with sharp edges may produce annoying collisions—and can also generate serious nerve and vein compression, most likely in your arms or wrists.

- A cluttered desk, especially with small, inconvenient storage areas, can force you to contort your body to retrieve materials.

Steps to Take

- Approach one-size-fits-all workstations with caution. Different bodies require different heights. Most people need to adjust their work-stations to fit them properly.

- Adjust your workstation so that your wrists float in a neutral position when you use the keyboard. If you raise your chair to attain this position and leave your feet dangling, use a footrest.

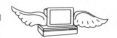

- Jobs have different space and height requirements—a graphic artist may require much more flat space than a data-entry clerk. Analyze your work, note the different positions required for each major task, then make sure your workspace fits your chores. Don't forget to reserve space for storage and telephone.

- Your primary work area should contain necessary materials well within easy reach. Store frequently needed materials close by, within an arm's length if possible. Don't place something so it requires you to stretch too far—better to get up and walk.

- To make space on your desk, see if you can move the main box of your computer out of your way, perhaps onto the floor (but make sure you aren't blocking its ventilation and causing it to overheat).

- You might be better off with a desk that has adjustable-height surfaces to accommodate different tasks or various postures you may adopt throughout the day. If so, make sure your chair adjusts to the various work surface heights and nestles close enough.

Keyboard Holders

- Keyboard holders can provide a simple solution for desks that are the wrong height—if you have the right holder and use it correctly.

- A simple pullout tray may be sufficient for your work, but make sure it places the keyboard at the height *you* need.

- Keyboard holders on cantilevered arms offer more adjustments; the best can be positioned above the desk surface as well as below, and don't bounce.

- If you use a mouse, make sure your keyboard holder provides ample room to hold it next to your keyboard. Reaching past the keyboard holder to use a mouse on the desk can place you in stressful positions.

- Keyboard holders aren't for everyone—some people find there is no place for writing materials when using them.

Stand Up, Sit Down Solution

- Intensive computer users may benefit from a workstation which adjusts to a standing configuration. When Pacific Bell acquired a few standing workstations for their directory assistance operators, they proved so popular that, to handle demand, operators were limited to 30-minute shifts.

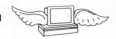

15. Key Craft

The standard QWERTY keyboard layout was adopted in the 1870s.

■ ■ ■

A combination of the right equipment combined with low stress positioning and good typing technique may help to reduce injury.

Keyboard Essentials

- A detachable keyboard helps you work in different comfortable positions. You may need an extra-long keyboard cord.

- A thin profile keeps the keys lower, making it more likely you can adjust your chair and desk correctly to keep your forearms parallel to the floor or tilted slightly up. A thin profile also keeps you from having to bend your wrists back to type.

- An adjustable angle helps you ensure that your wrists are flat and comfortable while you type.

- Scooped key tops encourage your fingers to remain in the correct positions.

- Moderate keystroke pressure pays various benefits. Too firm an action requires extra force. Too sensitive an action can produce input errors and hand tension.

- Key spacing and layout should help your fingers rest comfortably without crowding. For those with larger hands, the keyboards of some portable computers may seem awkward. Layout should be familiar, and frequently used side keys (Shift, Return, and so forth) should be close to the main keys.

- Tactile or aural feedback indicating when a keystroke is made helps you type. You'd miss it if it weren't there.

Steps to Take

- **Adjust your workstation** so your wrists are flat—not tilting up—while your fingers float over your keyboard and your forearms lie relatively parallel with the floor. Most desks are too high. Some experts suggest tilting the keyboard slightly away from you—propping up the front—to help level the wrists.

- **Consider a wrist rest.** Many people find that wrist rests help keep wrists and hands parallel to the keyboard. Many experts suggest you

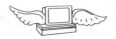

should keep your wrists "floating" while you type, and use the pad to give your wrists a comfortable resting place between typing. Wrist rests should be thick and padded, and sit even with the keyboard (although some people prefer slightly higher), not below it. Try out wrist rests to make sure they fit your equipment.

- **Easy does it.** Use macros to decrease the amount of keying you do. Take breaks from constant keyboard use. See page 28.

Good Typing Technique

Even the most well-designed and configured equipment may not protect you from injury if you don't use good typing technique. It's easy to fall into bad habits, so try to be aware of how you position yourself when you type.

- **Float hands and wrists.** Use the larger muscles of your arms to position your hands to help reduce stress on the smaller muscles in your fingers. Use wrist rests and chair arms for support when you are *not* typing. Make sure your arms or wrists don't jab into any hard or sharp edges.

- **Keep wrists neutral.** Don't bend your hands up (extension) or out (ulnar deviation) from your wrists. Ulnar deviation can be difficult to avoid, especially for larger people. Tip: try to be aware of your wrist position while typing, especially when hitting the Enter key.

- **Position fingers correctly.** Don't hold your fingers in awkward positions: crimped, stretched, or crumpled. Maintain neutral wrist position and arc fingers on a gentle, even curve.

- **Type lightly.** Studies show that most people hit the keys much harder than necessary, although it isn't known if this causes injury. To reduce impact on the fingers and hands, don't lift your hands far above the keyboard and bang your fingers down; instead keep a low hand position and "drop" your fingers.

- **Keep relaxed.** Maintain good posture without tensing the muscles in your arms, fingers, neck, or back. Don't press your elbows in tight to your body.

Resources

The HAND Book. Stephanie Brown (New York: Ergonome, 1993). An engaging and helpful book on how to type, written by a former piano instructor.

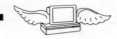

16. Avoid Mouse Traps

*The world's mouse population
is estimated at 60 million.*

■ ■ ■

Are mice, trackballs, and other pointing devices less painful to use than keyboards? Which has the fewest risks? No one knows. There is just not enough research into the physiological effects of prolonged pointing-device use to state many risks definitively.

Points to Remember

Dr. David Rempel, Director of the Ergonomics Laboratory at the University of California at Berkeley and San Francisco, suggests four ways to more safely move your mouse. Consider using these tips with other pointing devices as well.

■ Maintain a neutral wrist position.

■ Vary hand position throughout the day.

■ Don't press your hand into any hard edges.

■ Don't use force while clicking or dragging.

Add these tips, as well:

■ Let go of the pointing device when you aren't using it, to allow your hand and arm to relax.

■ Don't grip the device with too much force—a bad habit many mouse users fall into. Don't keep your arm constantly tensed while using the device, as this can tire the muscles and lead to injury.

■ Make sure you can operate your pointing device without stretching your arm or putting your body into awkward positions.

■ Watch out for keyboard trays that leave too little room for a mouse or tablet, forcing you to put the device where it's difficult to reach.

What Hurts?

If you think repeated button clicking gives you pain:

■ Try using keystrokes to replace clicking.

■ Try switching pointing device hands (but be aware that you may develop the same problems you had on the other limb).

■ Try either a foot pedal or mouse that requires less button force, but try it out before you buy it to see if it fits your body.

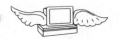

If repeated continual dragging seems to be your problem:

■ Try a drag-lock feature, which holds a "mouse-down" condition without continual pressure on the button. This may be a feature available with your mouse/software combination, or available as an inexpensive software addition.

If you find yourself moving the mouse long distances:

■ You might want to increase the mouse speed setting to reduce move-ment, but be vigilant for increased muscle tension.

If you experience shoulder soreness:

■ Consider switching to a trackball or switching to different size of device.

To reduce pain in the ring or little fingers:

■ Small hands may need to switch to a smaller device (like the original Microsoft Mouse), while large hands may benefit from a three-button device which is necessarily wider.

■ Consider a wrist rest to reduce wrist and finger extension. If you float your hands over your pointing device, try resting your fingers gently on it—you may reduce some of the load on the tendons at the elbow.

If you find yourself not moving the mouse with your arm:

■ Try changing the mouse speed and moving the mouse more with your arm—but watch out for shoulder pain!

Trackball Tips & Tricks

■ Most trackball designs promote wrist extension (bending the wrist upward). Placing a foam pad in front of the trackball may help.

■ Don't switch to a trackball and use it intensively right away. Gradually work these muscles into shape to avoid stressing them.

■ Make sure your thumb doesn't get sore from the trackball, and avoid devices that require you to move the ball with your thumb.

■ Most trackballs also have a drag-lock capability. Try it.

■ You might want to try out devices with variable tracking speeds, or alternative devices like touch pads.

Resource

Pointing Device Summary Document, Pete Johnson. The most current and comprehensive information on pointing devices. See page 72.

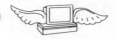

17. Light Fantastic

*In one study only 10% of New York City offices
had good visual environments for computers.*

■ ■ ■

Do you notice reflections in your screen before it's turned on? While
sitting at your workstation, does shielding your eyes make you feel
better? Reflections and bright lights can make monitors difficult to see.
You and your manager can take a number of easy steps (many of them at
no cost) to make your workplace easier on the eyes.

Common Office Lighting Hazards

■ Excessively bright general lighting

■ Bright areas in the field of vision

■ Glare on walls and surfaces

■ Reflections on screen

Lighting Principles

■ The main light sources in your office should be balanced with the
brightness of your screen. Traditionally, offices have been brightly lit
for working with paper—too bright for many computer monitors.

■ What you look at (the screen, reading material, keyboard, and so on)
should be of similar brightness; there should be no "hot spots" of light
noticeable behind or around the screen.

Steps to Take

Reduce major light sources so they don't overpower your screen.

■ You can easily reduce the intensity of fluorescent banks by removing
some of the tubes.

■ When switching off fluorescent lights makes the office too dark, use an
incandescent or halogen floor lamp with variable brightness control
that bounces light off the ceiling or walls, producing a soft effect.

■ Light sources behind and above you may need to be louvered, baffled,
repositioned, turned off, or otherwise modified to kill reflections. A
large plant can be positioned to block bright lights.

■ Daylight can brighten offices so monitors are nearly impossible to see.
Reduce daylight with blinds, partitions, or tinted windows. Daylight
varies, so make adjustments throughout the day.

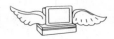

Match the brightnesses around you.

■ As a general rule, keep any bright light sources as far away from the field of vision as possible.

■ Office walls may be too light or their glossiness may produce shiny reflections. Painting walls a neutral color can decrease their brightness. Flat-finish paint and fabric-treated walls cut glare.

■ If bright spots in the field of vision can't be controlled, you may be able to shift your workstation into a more favorable position.

Reduce reflections in your screen.

■ Switching from a dark to light screen background may mask reflections. But be aware that sometimes less noticeable reflections still interfere with your seeing the screen clearly.

■ Glare shields or hoods may be great at preventing reflections, but they aren't universal cures for lighting problems. See page 52.

Use task lights with caution.

■ Task lights can provide ample light in a small area, perfect for lighting documents at the computer when the ambient light level is low. But task lights are often too bright—make sure yours isn't.

■ Position task lights carefully, so they don't throw bright light directly into your eyes.

Notes for Managers

The perfect lighting design is elastic and accessible—it must adjust to the changing conditions of the office environment and the different needs of its inhabitants.

■ The light surrounding a workstation often changes. Office lights go on and off, and daylight varies throughout the day. Lighting must be adjustable enough to meet these changing conditions.

■ Lighting adjustment should be in the hands of the people who need it. Lighting requirements vary among individuals depending on age, workstation geography, computer screen, and job type.

Resources

Illuminating Engineering Society of North America. 120 Wall Street, 17th floor, New York, NY 10005. (212) 248-5000. Publishes *Lighting for Offices Containing Computer Visual Display Terminals* (1989) for $35 plus $3 shipping.

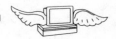

18. Mind Your Monitor

If not set up and used properly, even the best monitor can give you eyestrain.

■ ■ ■

Computer monitors may be miracles of engineering, but they still need your periodic attention and adjustment to deliver an image that's easy on your eyes.

Screen Hazards to Watch For

■ Monitors attract dust—color monitors generally attract more dust than monochrome.

■ Brightness can vary dramatically from one monitor to another. Dim screens make glare more obtrusive, and produce a low-contrast image; both make the eye work harder.

■ Most screens are treated in some manner to reduce their reflective properties. However, all surface treatments represent compromises: some reduce brightness, contrast, and sharpness, others exaggerate dirt—especially oily dirt such as fingerprints.

Operator Errors

Display choices that you make can affect screen legibility and your reading efficiency.

■ Small type is hard to see; some monitors may not have sufficient resolution to display smaller font sizes adequately. Type that is too large slows down your reading, and makes you scroll around more within a document. Choose a type height that's clear and comfortable to see.

■ Some people get a color monitor and go Hollywood, making their type green, the background red, and their boldface blue. Although the judicious use of color can make images clearer, it's hard to concentrate on many different colors simultaneously; adjacent areas of red and blue are particularly difficult to focus on. Choose colors that will give good contrast between the letters and their background.

■ An excessive alteration of the monitor's position may reduce reflections and glare but still cause eyestrain by making the image too difficult to see. Positioning the monitor off to one side so that you must twist to see it may seriously strain your back or neck.

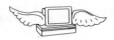

Steps You Can Take

- **Position your monitor** more than 18" (45 cm) from your eyes allowing for a downward gaze angle to all parts of the screen. Traditional advice placed the top of the screen at eye height, but some experts now suggest that lower may be better. But beware of introducing new reflections.

- **Clean your screen**—it's the easiest way to increase your monitor's performance. A clean screen is brighter and produces more contrast. Clean your screen before dust becomes noticeable.

- **Use a nonscratching towel** (available from many computer stores and catalogs) moistened with glass cleaner (or a weak solution of soap and water), followed by a damp towel rinse and a wipe clean. **Careful:** Some coatings and plastic screens scratch easily; attempting to clean these could damage them and render them worse than before. Always follow the manufacturer's cleaning instructions.

- **Turn up the brightness** of your monitor if the light level in your office is high and cannot easily be controlled. But watch out for the trade-off between brightness and sharpness: some monitors can be adjusted so brightly that their image becomes fuzzy.

- **Consider a glare filter** if you have reflections in your screen you can't control. Glare filters can sometimes magically improve the appearance of your display—but can also make an image worse.

- **Consider a hood** as a simple and inexpensive solution to reflections in the screen. Although available from manufacturers, it can be constructed out of cardboard and tape with a minimum of skill. Black cardboard with a matte finish is best.

White or Black Background?

- Black characters on a white background are easier to see than vice versa: people are used to viewing printed text in that form, and a large white field reduces the effect of screen reflections.

- **White background notes:** When displaying large areas of white, some monitors actually dim slightly and flicker is more noticeable. Try changing the background to a light green or blue, but maintain a high contrast between the background and foreground.

- **Dark background notes:** Be sure to minimize reflections in the screen through lighting control and monitor positioning—and, yes, some people even resort to wearing a dark shirt so they won't see themselves reflected in the screen.

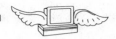

19. Image Quality

*Flickering and blurry screens can cause the eyes
to work too hard to focus, resulting in eyestrain.*

■ ■ ■

Even when placed in a perfect visual environment, the image quality of monitors varies widely, and it can have a big impact on your comfort level. There are fixes, but expert help may be required.

Flicker and Blur

- As screens age, image quality degrades and brightness becomes less uniform, often without your noticing. This decline in image quality can cause eyestrain.

- Flickering screens—even if barely perceptible to the eye—cause the eye to continually readjust, leading to fatigue and headaches. About 10% of people are particularly sensitive to flicker.

- Screen focus is a subjective quality, yet it relates directly to a monitor's legibility. Eyestrain can result as the eye continually refocuses on a blurry image in a vain attempt to make it clear.

- Occasionally, external magnetic fields may degrade the image of your monitor—introducing odd colors and "bending" the image in uncomfortable ways.

Image Quality Fixes

- **If you are bothered by screen flicker,** a technician may be able to adjust your monitor's vertical refresh rate to a higher, less noticeable, value. A vertical refresh rate above 70 Hz produces a flicker-free picture for most viewers (in larger or brighter screens, flicker is more apparent). However, make sure the higher rate doesn't significantly decrease the sharpness of the image.

- **If your monitor seems fuzzy,** have it adjusted. (Simple shop adjustments usually cost between $50 and $100.) **Warning:** Don't try to adjust internal controls yourself; the voltages can be lethal, even after the monitor has been off for a while.

- **If your monitor has a color shift** on one of its sides or corners, especially toward pink or blue, turn it off and back on. Your monitor may have needed to be demagnetized (*degaussed* is the technical term). Most screens automatically degauss when you turn them off and then

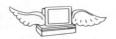

on again, although some monitors have a separate push button degaussing feature. If degaussing doesn't work, seek expert assistance.

- **If your monitor dances the hula**, flickers, swims, or has weird colored blotches, an external magnetic field may be influencing it. Try moving objects like electric pencil sharpeners or speakers away from the monitor. If that doesn't work, call an expert—a bad power supply or nearby power lines may be the culprit.

In the Market for a Monitor?

- Choose a combination of monitor and graphics board that produce a stable, flicker-free image. Look for a high "refresh rate" (above 75 Hz), a "non-interlaced" display mode, and resolution settings that result in a clear image without excessively small interface elements.

- Check out magazine reviews of monitors, but then see which looks best to you by making side-by-side comparisons of your favorites in computer stores.

- Find a monitor that can make small type, like 5-point, sharp and legible. That's a good indication it can display 12-point type (a normal size for much work) extremely clearly.

- Examine the monitor's spec sheet and determine the dot pitch. Dot pitch represents (more or less) the distance between each of the red, green, and blue phosphor clusters that produce your screen's image. Generally, the smaller the dot pitch, the more precise the image. A monitor with a dot pitch of .28 mm or less is capable of producing a sharp image.

- Look for controls that are accessible and easy to use. Some monitors can remember different user settings—a bonus if your office lighting conditions vary.

Resources

DisplayMate. Sonera Technologies, P.O. Box 565, Rumson, NJ 07760. (800) 932-6323. The most advanced diagnostic testing software for monitors. $149.

TCO (The Swedish Confederation of Professional Employees). 150 N. Michigan Avenue, Suite 1200, Chicago, IL 60601-7594. (312) 781-6223. Fax (312) 346-0683. Certifies equipment meeting its ergonomic and radiation standard for desktop computers. Offers book explaining monitor facts ($27). Sells kits to help evaluate monitors ($10) and software ($100 with disk).

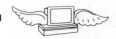

20. Glare Filters

A glare filter can be a great step forward in making your monitor's image clear and legible.

■ ■ ■

Glare filters increase your screen's contrast by reducing the reflected glare more than the emitted light. Reflected light passes through the filter twice, while light emitted by the monitor passes through only once. Glare filters often work wonders on dark background monitors.

Glaring truths

■ Some filters are electrically conductive and designed to be grounded, reducing the monitor's attraction of dust.

■ It is best to try a filter to make sure it is effective for your work area (find one with a money-back guarantee). If the filter makes the monitor harder to see, ditch it.

■ The American Optometric Association evaluates and approves glare screens. An AOA Seal of Acceptance is one indicator of a glare filter's quality and effectiveness.

Hard filters

■ Most hard filters carry anti-reflective coatings and a tint or polarization application to increase contrast. In certain situations, a polarized filter's effectiveness can be extraordinary.

■ A hard filter can trap dust, and some create more reflection problems than they solve. Generally, the closer they are mounted to the screen (some adhere to it) the better. Optical purity is a must, and can be lacking, particularly in the plastic models.

Mesh filters

■ Mesh filters act as a dark, matte scrim, absorbing the light hitting the screen at an angle. They are particularly effective when there is a bright light reflecting directly off the screen.

■ On the down side, mesh filters can: partially obscure the screen image, reflect light from certain angles, and create moiré patterns.

Resource

American Optometric Association. 243 North Lindbergh Blvd., St. Louis, MO 63141. (314) 991-4100. Certifies quality glare filters.

ALL THE
REST

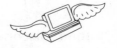

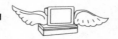

21. Fields & Beams

We live in an electrical society; we are exposed to electromagnetic energy almost everywhere.

■■■

We don't think anyone should tell you that the electromagnetic energy generated by computers is safe—or is dangerous. No one knows for sure. But we do think you should have an idea of what this "radiation" really is, and why some scientists believe it's harmless, while others want to investigate its potential danger. So let's dispel some myths and see what easy steps you can take to reduce exposure to electromagnetic energy, if you wish to.

Common Misconceptions

Computer monitors emit X-rays.

Computer monitors, like televisions, produce X-rays, a form of electro-magnetic energy that can harm living tissue. But not to worry: these X-rays are contained inside the tube, so they pose no health threat. Devices that claim to block dangerous X-rays emitted by your monitor are a waste of money.

Computer monitors cause cancer.

No reputable scientist would suggest there's incontrovertible evidence that proves monitors cause cancer or other serious health effects. Some scientists think the evidence linking a few types of cancers to electro-magnetic energy of extremely low frequencies (ELF) warrants more research. Some also suggest there's no harm in reducing your exposure to electromagnetic energy as long as it's easy to do so.

You can prevent your exposure to electromagnetic energy.

Not unless you live in a deep cave, since sunlight and radio waves are forms of electromagnetic energy. Electrical power from wiring, lights, and equipment (including computer equipment) radiates electromag-netic energy throughout businesses, homes, and beyond.

All office equipment creates the same type of electromagnetic energy.

Different types of electronic equipment produce electromagnetic energy with different characteristics. Some people speculate that the type of energy produced by computer monitors may be particularly harmful, but so far there is little evidence to support this view.

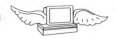

Did You Know?

- The term radiation is routinely used as a label for different forms of energy—from *electromagnetic energy* (which includes the energy produced by computers) to gamma rays (a stream of subatomic particles).

- Computers, like most electrical equipment, produce electromagnetic energy as electromagnetic *fields* and electromagnetic *radiation*. One difference between these is that when you turn off the electromagnetic source, the radiation that had been produced continues to move out through space (it is "radiated"), whereas the field collapses into the source.

- It turns out that at the low frequencies generated by computers, the electromagnetic fields (EMFs) are stronger than the radiation.

- It also turns out that monitors produce both *electric* fields and *magnetic* fields. Electric fields can be shielded very easily. Magnetic fields are difficult to shield, but monitor manufacturers can engineer monitors so the magnetic fields outside them are very low. Some experts who consider that electromagnetic energy from computers might be a health threat speculate that the magnetic fields might be the cause.

Steps to Take

The first steps:

- **Stay positive.** Some experts say that stressing out over EMF is much more likely to hurt you than any threat posed by the fields. If you think fields are dangerous, then follow the reasonable precautions outlined below.

- **Be a smart computer consumer.** Unscrupulous marketers use the fear about EMFs and the complexity of the issues to sell ineffective and sometimes dangerous products. Don't buy lead shields. Scrutinize the claims of glare screens that supposedly block EMFs; they may only shield the electric fields, not the magnetic fields that some researchers are most concerned about.

Reasonable precautions:

- **Use a monitor that conforms to MPRII or TCO guidelines.** Check for them on your monitor's specifications sheet. These low-EMF guidelines are not proven safe, but the guidelines do stipulate lower fields than those emitted by most older monitors. Almost all new monitors built in the U.S. meet the MPRII guidelines.

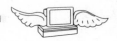

- **Stay an arm's length away from your screen.** Even with higher-emission monitors, staying an arm's length (about 30 inches or 75 cm) from the screen drops the EMFs to the background levels found in most offices. You may need to increase the size of objects on your screen (such as text) so you can see them at this distance.

- **Stay four feet (about 1.2 meters) away from the back and the sides of monitors.** Fields can be stronger there. And be aware that walls and partitions don't block these fields.

- **Turn your monitor off when you're not using it.** It's easy to reduce most of your exposure to the monitor's EMF—*and save electricity*—by just turning your monitor off. According to the Environmental Protection Agency (EPA), 80% of the time a monitor is operating, it isn't being viewed. Many new computers and monitors comply with the EPA's Energy Star program, automatically powering down or going to a lower-power state when not in use.

- **Consult with your doctor if you are pregnant.** Some women have limited their time on the computer while pregnant, or trying to become pregnant, but few studies suggest this is necessary. If you are concerned, check with your doctor. See page 57.

- **Consider other EMF sources.** If you are worried about EMFs, it may not make sense to reduce exposure to your monitor while there are much more potent EMF emitters in your environment. However, it's questionable how much you can practically reduce your exposure, and what this reduction might mean to your health.

- **The worst offenders.** In the home, older electric blankets may expose you to the most EMFs, as they are close to the body for long periods of time. Many electric shavers, can openers, and power tools generate strong EMFs, and are operated near your body (though for shorter periods). In the office, desk lamps and some laser printers and photocopiers generate significant EMFs.

Resource

The best source we've found on electromagnetic fields and computers is the industry newsletter *VDT NEWS*—but it's expensive. You might be able to find it at a large public or university library. *VDT NEWS*, PO Box 1799, Grand Central Station, New York, NY. 10163 (212) 517-2803.

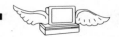

22. Great Expectations

*A few precautions can reduce dangers
to developing babies.*

■ ■ ■

Smoking, diet, chemicals, medications, garden work, exercise—it seems like nearly everything can potentially damage the health of a developing baby. So it wasn't surprising when about 15 years ago some researchers began suspecting that computer work might be added to the list.

Can working at a computer hurt your developing baby, or can it hurt you as a pregnant woman? Maybe, but probably not—especially if you take a few simple precautions.

Possible Threats to the Developing Child

Stress

- Psychological stress, a factor that's often associated with computerized offices, has been shown to be involved in negative pregnancy outcomes.

- People have different reactions to stressful situations. How much stress causes damage to a fetus varies considerably among women and situations.

Electromagnetic Fields

- Research has not proven a strong link between electromagnetic fields and miscarriage or birth defects.

- Although a few animal studies showed fetal damage resulting from magnetic fields, and a new epidemiological study suggested a link between extremely low frequency (ELF) fields and miscarriage, many other results have been negative.

- A recent British review of VDT pregnancy studies found no support for risk.

- A large Danish epidemiological study released in late 1992 found no correlation between miscarriage and computer use.

- In 1990, a NIOSH (National Institute of Occupational Safety and Health) study concluded that "the use of VDTs and exposure to the accompanying electromagnetic fields were not associated with an increased risk of spontaneous abortions."

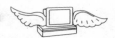

Possible Threats to the Mother

Fluid buildup

- Pregnancy causes fluid retention. That fact coupled with the tendency of pregnant women to be less active means that when they sit, they often experience a fluid buildup in their legs and feet.

- As a rule, sitting on the job seems to be good for your developing child. Those women who stand in fixed positions while they work (for example, hairdressers and dentists) have about twice as many premature births as those who sit on the job.

- However, women sitting in the constrained postures associated with computer work have not been specifically studied, so there may be more information for computer users in the future.

Carpal tunnel syndrome and De Quervain's Disease

- Up to 35% of pregnant women—whether they work on the computer or not—experience carpal tunnel syndrome (CTS) or De Quervain's disease (a tendon sheath disorder near the base of the thumb) during or immediately after pregnancy.

- These maladies may be due to swelling from increased fluid retention.

- Doctors don't know if computer work accelerates or aggravates CTS and De Quervain's disease, but some suggest it may.

- Normally, pregnancy-related CTS disappears immediately after the birth, and De Quervain's often subsides sometime after birth.

Steps to Take

- If you are pregnant or plan to get pregnant, tell your doctor about your work at the keyboard (she'll want to know anyway).

Stay cool.

- As a rule, you want to pay special attention to your psychological stress load during pregnancy.

- Make sure to discuss work-related stress with your doctor. For more ideas on stress magangement, see page 32.

Take EMF in stride.

- If you have had trouble conceiving or carrying a child to term, you may want to exercise additional caution regarding factors that may cause miscarriage.

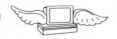

- Seek your doctor's advice, follow the well-known suggestions that have been proven to produce a healthy child, stay informed of the issues, and take sensible precautions if they ease your mind and help reduce your stress level. See page 32.

- Many women who have expressed concern about electromagnetic fields have negotiated with their employers for reduced time at the computer, for transfer to another job while pregnant, or for purchase of a low-emission monitor.

- Don't use a lead apron, which does nothing to block these fields, but poses a risk to your fetus by pressing on it.

Avoid fluid buildup.

- Fluid buildup discomfort can be minimized if you remember not to sit for long periods; get up and stretch and move.

- If the condition continues to bother you, consider a 20-minute rest in the afternoon lying on your left side, which can promote circulation and reduce the buildup of fluid.

- Off the job, swim, walk, or partake of other moderate exercise to promote good circulation.

Pay attention to your hands and wrists.

- If you believe you may be developing a cumulative trauma disorder, be sure to inform your doctor, and don't forget to remind her about the time you spend at the computer.

- Because of their transitory nature, both CTS and De Quervain's may be treated with splints; if this is not effective, doctors may prescribe steroid injections (after the baby is weaned) or surgery.

- Prudence suggests that you seek a second opinion before resorting to surgery. See page 60.

Resources

VDT NEWS. PO Box 1799, Grand Central Station, New York, NY 10163. (212) 517-2803. Thorough but expensive newsletter on the entire range of computer-health issues.

9to5, National Association of Working Women. (414) 274-0925. Organization focuses on several issues affecting office workers, particularly those affecting women, including reproductive risks.

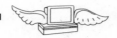

23. The Right Doctor

If you think you have a CTD, have it checked out immediately by as good a doctor as you can find.

■ ■ ■

"How do you find the right doctor?" No other question can invoke as much dismay in a sufferer of a cumulative trauma disorder (CTD). Many people with computer-related CTDs have to grope their way through the medical system—often being incorrectly or inadequately diagnosed and treated—before they find someone who can give them the proper care. Many others are still looking.

Doctors experienced in workplace CTDs are more likely to give you the best care; doctors in certain specialties are more likely to have that experience. You can narrow your search and then question the doctor and assess if he or she is right for you. When in doubt, ask about experience, training, and certification.

Which Specialties?

A doctor with workplace CTD experience can specialize in a number of different areas. Here's a rundown:

- **Occupational medicine specialists** are trained to make a connection between an injury and the workplace. Those that are board-certified in occupational medicine have had training in CTD-related injuries, but some of these doctors work principally in areas like toxicology.

- **Physical medicine specialists** are experts in the rehabilitative aspects of medicine; they are well versed in soft-tissue musculoskeletal problems. Board certification in physical medicine is highly desirable.

- **Orthopedic surgery specialists** are more apt to advise a significant course of nonsurgical treatment than are other types of surgeons. If you have hand or wrist pain, make sure the orthopedist treats hand injuries, which is a subspecialty of orthopedics.

- Few **family practitioners, general practitioners, and internists** possess much experience in this small realm of disorders. It is not unknown for less experienced doctors to make diagnoses of carpal tunnel syndrome and recommend splints or surgery when carpal tunnel syndrome isn't the real problem. A good family practitioner unfamiliar in this area will refer you to the right specialist.

- **Other health care professionals**—physical therapists, occupational therapists, recreational therapists, some specialty nurses, and some

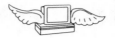

specialty psychologists, to name a few—may also be experienced with CTDs. Knowledge is the key. Some sufferers have found help from practitioners of other schools of health care, including chiropractors, acupuncturists, and massage therapists.

First Steps to Finding the Right Doctor

Get recommendations.

- Your goal is straightforward: find a doctor who has successfully treated conditions similar to yours.

- Make a list of as many CTD sufferers as you can; ask in your office, network, query your friends. Then ask your contacts if they have found good doctors. The emphatic affirmatives are worth following up.

- In a few geographical areas there are support groups and agencies that keep names of knowledgeable workplace-CTD physicians.

Check out hospitals and clinics.

- If you don't get a strong recommendation, you're on your own; start with the Yellow Pages.

- Many hospitals have occupational and physical medicine clinics; teaching hospitals associated with universities often have experienced and interested doctors who are versed in the latest procedures.

- You might also find a good doctor at a sports medicine clinic.

- Once you find a clinic, call and ask for the doctor who handles the most cases involving workplace CTDs. If the front desk can't help, ask to speak with a nurse.

Check Your Doctor Out

You can phone the doctor and ask the following questions as a preliminary screening method. If you cannot talk to the doctor within a few days, you may want to try someone else. How the doctor answers your questions is just as important as what she says.

- **What kinds of treatment do you offer for cumulative trauma disorders?** By the way the doctor answers, you can get an idea if she is primarily surgical or nonsurgical. You'll probably want to try nonsurgical treatment before resorting to surgery.

- **Do you often suggest workplace intervention?** You want a doctor who considers the workplace in her diagnoses and is willing to suggest changes in your workplace.

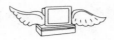

- **How many work-related CTD cases do you treat?** Someone in a specialty CTD clinic may see four people a day with these kinds of problems; a hand surgeon probably sees more than that.

- **Do you believe that cumulative trauma disorders exist and are related to work?** Some doctors don't believe CTDs exist, but may not give you an honest answer. Accept a cautious answer—it's justified—but be leery of a hostile or evasive one.

- **Do you handle workers' compensation cases?** If you are covered by workers' compensation, you need a doctor who will accept such cases. Many doctors find the paperwork and fee structure onerous.

Resources

A number of organizations will help you find a competent doctor.

Finding a health care professional. These organizations may be able to suggest clinics or physicians in your area that are experienced in treating workplace CTDs.

- **American Academy of Physical Medicine & Rehabilitation.** (312) 922-9366. This organization will supply names of physical medicine specialists in your area.

- **American Occupational Medical Association (AOMA).** (708) 228-6850. Will supply names of occupational medicine specialists in your area. Contact Public Relations or Education.

- **Office Technology Education Project.** (617) 776-2777. Located in Massachusetts.

- **Committees for Occupational Safety and Health (COSH)** and affiliated organizations. Found in most states.

Checking competence. These organizations may help you research a particular doctor's competence.

- **American Board of Medical Specialties (ABMS)** certification line. (800) 776-2378. This nonprofit organization provides at no charge information about doctors who are board-certified in a specialty, including the date that they were certified and for what specialties.

- **Public Citizen Health Research Group.** (202) 833-3000. Publishes list of doctors who have been disciplined by state boards. You can order the chapter for your state for about $10.

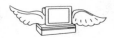

24. A Good Examination

You must be your own health advocate.

■ ■ ■

If your doctor doesn't get a complete picture on the initial evaluation, she probably never will. You can improve your chances of an accurate diagnosis and a satisfying office visit with a few easy steps.

What to Bring to the Exam

Know your symptoms—precisely determine and write down what feels or looks wrong:

- Make sure you note when the problem started, how it may have changed, and what may aggravate the pain.
- See if you can reproduce the symptoms by putting your body in certain positions. Don't hurt yourself doing this!

Write down various aspects of your job including:

- How long you sit at the computer, making repetitive motions.
- What positions you work in, especially any that seem awkward.
- If you are under deadline pressures or other psychosocial stress.
- If any of your co-workers have been diagnosed with CTDs.
- Your workstation setup.

Many people benefit from taking a friend or relative to the initial examination:

- Besides providing moral support, a friend can make sure you ask all your questions.
- Another set of ears and someone to discuss the interview with can be especially helpful; patients often don't remember important remarks the doctor makes during the examination.

Expect an adequate examination.

The doctor needs to devote enough time to make an adequate examination and establish a relationship with you.

On the first visit to the doctor you should be asked questions similar to the following:

- How did it start?
- What makes it worse?

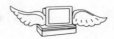

- What makes it better?
- What things at work aggravate it?
- What things outside of work aggravate it?

Also during the exam:

- The doctor should make a complete exploration of all your symptoms.

- If your doctor doesn't look at and feel the neck and shoulder region, you should demand it. A thorough exam from the neck down is essential for proper diagnosis.

- Feel free to ask questions and make sure you understand the answers. If something is unclear, ask, ask, and ask again.

- Take notes so you can review the examination at your leisure.

After the visit:

- If you feel you received a good examination from a good doctor, follow her advice. You are the active partner in returning yourself to good health.

- You may be asked to return to work. Many doctors familiar with computer injury realize that intervention in the workplace can aid in recovery, and stopping work may be detrimental to healing in many situations.

- However, chronic CTD sufferers counsel you should be wary if you are only medicated and sent back to work, or if the doctor says, "It will go away in a couple of weeks; just wear these splints."

- If you don't feel like the doctor has examined you fully or taken a good history, consider finding another doctor.

Resources

Get Well, Stay Well: The Successful Patient's Handbook. Barry Gordon, M.D. (New York: Dembner Books, 1988). A blunt yet revealing aid for dealing with doctors and the medical system. Particularly insightful in the preparations you can make that help the doctor do the best job.

Smart Questions to Ask Your Doctor. Dorothy Leeds (New York: Harper Paperbacks, 1992). Useful compendium of questions to ask doctors, to improve your chances of receiving the best care.

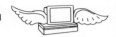

25. Medications

All pain relievers have possible side effects.

■ ■ ■

Sometimes computer work causes pain. Headache, eyestrain, and cumulative trauma disorders may have you reaching for over-the-counter medications. In more extreme cases, you may find relief with medications only available with a doctor's prescription.

Medications can be a valuable and welcome relief for computer-induced pain, but they must be used wisely. Many are powerful drugs with potentially serious side effects. And unless you use them rarely, most medications represent only a temporary or partial solution for a computer-related health problem.

Don't Take These Lightly

- All of the drugs listed in this chapter can have serious side effects. In most cases these problems are rare, but since the list is as long as your arm, it is only practical to list a smattering of them. These drugs can be potent, so use them with good sense.

- Follow your doctor's instructions and any directions that come with the medication. If you have a question about medication, ask a pharmacist or your doctor.

- If you are pregnant, nursing, taking a prescription drug, or on a diet prescribed by your doctor (low-salt, low-sugar), check with your doctor before taking any over-the-counter pain relievers.

- If you find yourself taking a pain reliever day after day without a doctor's supervision, tell your doctor.

Over-the-Counter Pain Relievers

It is a common misconception that drugs are sold over the counter because they are safe and not as potent as prescription medications. These pain relievers can be so effective they are often prescribed by doctors.

NSAIDs (Aspirin, Ibuprofen)

The nonsteroidal, anti-inflammatory drugs (NSAIDs) represent some of the most successful drugs available. They are inexpensive, yet can effectively relieve pain, inflammation, and swelling.

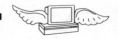

- If you find you can't tolerate one NSAID, there is sufficient variety available that another may work for you.

- Many people get upset stomachs (and a few can develop ulcers) from taking NSAIDs; aspirin is considered slightly worse than ibuprofen in this regard.

- To ease stomach irritation, take these medications at mealtime or with a glass of milk, or dissolve the tablet in a glass of water.

- Buffered aspirin, touted to be easier on the stomach than normal aspirin, actually isn't.

- Coated aspirin does cause less stomach irritation, but instead can irritate the lower intestine and takes longer to work.

Acetaminophen (Anacin-3, Tylenol)

- If you can't tolerate NSAIDs, then acetaminophen is often the over-the-counter pain reliever of choice. It is easier on the stomach than NSAIDs, but not completely benign, so you may want to take it at mealtimes or with milk.

- Because of the potential for liver damage, you shouldn't take acetaminophen for over 10 days without a doctor's approval.

- Think twice about drinking alcohol while taking acetaminophen (especially if you regularly drink alcohol), as you might be increasing your risk of liver damage.

- And taking high doses of vitamin C prevents your body from excreting acetaminophen, which could lead to liver and kidney damage.

Mind over Pain

Drugs are not the only method of controlling pain. Many people are able to reduce their pain through relaxation exercises and pain-control techniques. If you can't or don't want to take medications, ask your doctor for alternatives.

Resources

The Aspirin Handbook: A User's Guide to the Breakthrough Drug of the 90s. Joe Graedon, Tom Ferguson, and Teresa Graedon (New York: Bantam Books, 1993).

The American Medical Association Guide to Prescription and Over-the-Counter Drugs. Charles B. Clayman, editor (New York: Random House, 1988).

WHERE
ELSE TO
TURN

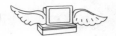

Books & Pamphlets

■ ■ ■

Zap! How your computer can hurt you—and what you can do about it, Don
Sellers (Berkeley, CA: Peachpit Press, 1994). *25 Steps to Safe Computing* was based
on *Zap!*, a comprehensive, accessible handbook on computer-related injuries.

20/20: A Total Guide to Improving Your Vision and Preventing Eye Disease.
Mitchell H. Friedlaender & Stef Donev (Emmaus, PA: Rodale Press, 1991).

***American National Standard for Human Factors Engineering of Visual Display
Terminal Workstations.*** Human Factors Society, Inc. (*see* Organizations).
Includes specifications of safe chair design.

***The American Medical Association Guide To Prescription And Over-The-
Counter Drugs.*** Charles B. Clayman, editor (New York: Random House, 1988).
Solid, comprehensive source for drug information.

The Aspirin Handbook: A User's Guide to the Breakthrough Drug of the 90s. Joe
Graedon, Tom Ferguson, and Teresa Graedon (New York: Bantam Books, 1993).
Everything you wanted to know (and more) about aspirin and other types of
pain relievers.

Basic Stuff: A Survival Guide to Workers' Compensation. Dorsey Hamilton.
Compensation Alert, 843 2nd St., Santa Rosa, CA 95404. (707) 545-2266. $12
including shipping and handling, considered as a tax-deductible contribution. A
worker-oriented guide to the California workers' compensation system.

The Best in Medicine. How and Where to Find the Best Health Care Available.
Herbert J. Dietrich and Virginia H. Biddle (New York: Harmony Books, 1990
revised edition). Authoritative guide to top hospitals and specialty clinics in the
United States. Includes section on rehabilitation clinics but not occupational-
medicine clinics.

Carpal Tunnel Syndrome: Evaluation, Treatment, and Prevention. Mark
Koniuch and John Palazzo (Thorofare, NJ: Slack Publishing, 1993).

Employee Burnout: America's Newest Epidemic (phone survey conducted in
1991) and ***Employee Burnout: Causes and Cures.*** Free pamphlet directed toward
companies measuring organizational stress. Includes stress test. Write to:
Northwestern National Life Insurance Company, PO Box 20, Route 6528,
Minneapolis, MN 55440.

Get Well, Stay Well: The Successful Patient's Handbook. Barry Gordon, M.D.
(New York: Dembner Books, 1988). A blunt yet revealing aid for dealing with
doctors and the medical system. Particularly insightful in the preparations you
can make that help the doctor do the best job.

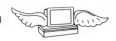

The HAND Book. Stephanie Brown. $19.95 plus shipping from: Ergonome, Inc., 145 West 96th Street, New York, NY 10025. (212) 222-9600. Fax (212) 222-6699. Illustrated volume on hand and arm injury prevention from a pianist. Includes hand-positioning poster.

Health Care USA. Jean Carper (New York: Prentice Hall, 1987). Lists superior hospitals and health institutions in the United States.

Healthy Computing: Risks and Remedies Every Computer User Needs To Know. Ronald Harwin (New York: Amacom, 1992).

Listen to Your Pain: The Active Person's Guide to Understanding, Identifying, and Treating Pain and Injury. Ben E. Benjamin (New York: Viking Press, 1984).

Repetitive Strain Injury: A Computer User's Guide. Emil Pascarelli, MD, and Deborah Quilter (New York: John Wiley & Sons, 1994). Solid book by clinician with over 20 years experience treating CTDs.

Sitting on the Job: How to Survive the Stresses of Sitting Down to Work. Scott Donkin; contributing editor Joseph Sweere (Boston: Houghton Mifflin Company, 1989).

Smart Questions To Ask Your Doctor. Dorothy Leeds (New York: Harper Paperbacks, 1992). Useful compendium of questions to ask doctors to improve your chances of receiving the best care.

Soft Tissue Pain and Disability. Rene Cailliet (Philadelphia: F.A. Davis, 1988) (2nd edition).

Stretch and Strengthen. Judy Alter (Boston: Houghton Mifflin, 1986).

Stretching. Bob Anderson (New York: Random House, 1980).

Treat Your Own Back. Robin McKenzie (Waikanae, New Zealand: Spinal Publications, 1988). Practical guide to back pain.

Treat Your Own Neck. Robin McKenzie (Waikanae, New Zealand: Spinal Publications, 1988). Practical guide to neck pain.

The Wellness Book: The Comprehensive Guide to Maintaining Health and Treating Stress-Related Illness. Herbert Benson, Eileen Stuart, and associates at the Mind/Body Medical Institute of the New England Deaconess Hospital and Harvard Medical School (New York: Simon and Schuster, 1993).

Workers' Compensation Claims Deskbook. Gwen Hampton (Glendale, CA: Workers' Compensation Co., 1993). Referred to as the bible of workers' compensation, and reportedly used by caseworkers in California. $92.00. The latest edition came out in August 1993. Workers' Compensation Company, PO Box 11448, Glendale, CA 91226. (818) 247-8224.

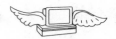

Organizations
■ ■ ■

9to5, National Association of Working Women. 238 West Wisconsin Ave., Suite 700, Milwaukee, WI 53203-2308. (414) 274-0925. 9to5 focuses on protecting the rights of office workers. They have a job problem hotline—(800) 522-0925—for people to call who are experiencing or witnessing work-related problems of any kind.

American Academy of Ophthalmology. PO Box 7424, San Francisco, CA 94120-7424. (415) 561-8500. Primarily a support organization for ophthalmologists, individuals can call to get individual copies of brochures on health issues related to the eye.

American Academy of Physical Medicine & Rehabilitation. (312) 922-9366. Will supply names of physical medicine specialists in your area.

American Board of Medical Specialties certification line, (800) 776-2378. This nonprofit organization provides free information about doctors who are board-certified in a specialty, including the date that they were certified and for what specialty or specialties (except in Alaska.)

American Occupational Medical Association (AOMA). 2340 South Arlington Heights Rd., Arlington Heights, IL 60005. (708) 228-6850. Will supply names of occupational medicine specialists in your area. Contact either Public Relations or Education department.

American Optometric Association. 243 North Lindbergh Blvd., St. Louis, MO 63141. (314) 991-4100. They distribute a pamphlet called *VDT User's Guide to Better Vision.* They also certify glare filters and will tell you over the telephone which filters have met their certification standards.

The Arthritis Foundation. PO Box 19000, Atlanta, GA 30326. (800) 283-7800 or (404) 872-7100. Provides information and materials, including a free brochure on back care and back pain. In Canada: The Arthritis Society, National Office, 250 Bloor Street E., Suite 901, Toronto, Ontario M4W 3P2. (416) 967-1414. Fax (416) 967-7171.

Association for Repetitive Motion Syndrome (ARMS). PO Box 514, Santa Rosa, CA 95402-05124. (707) 571-0397. This nonprofit organization provides information on repetitive strain injuries. Publishes newsletter. They accept calls from 10 am to 5 pm Pacific Time only.

Human Factors and Ergonomics Society. PO Box 1369, Santa Monica, CA 90406-1369. (310) 394-1811. Fax (310) 394-2410. They offer a directory of human factors and ergonomics consultants that is organized geographically and available for $35 to nonmembers or $20 to members. HFES also publishes papers including the ANSI standards on VDT workstations.

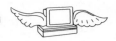

Job Accommodation Network. 918 Chestnut Ridge Rd., Suite 1, PO Box 6080, Morgantown, WV 26506-6080. (800) 526-7234 or (800) ADA-WORK or (304) 293-7186. This free service will supply information about the Americans with Disabilities Act to anyone who calls. The service, which offers advice on how to accommodate the disabled, is used primarily by employers, rehabilitation professionals, and people with disabilities. In Canada, call a Canadian-government-sponsored number: (800) 526-2262.

Labor Occupational Health Program. School of Public Health, University of California at Berkeley, 2515 Channing Way, 2nd Floor, Berkeley, CA 94720. (510) 642-5507. Nonprofit organization that provides job safety and health information, mainly to workers and the public. Maintains library and publishes educational material.

National Headache Foundation. 5252 N. Western Avenue, Chicago, Illinois 60625. (312) 878-7715. Nonprofit organization that provides general, up-to-date information about headaches. To receive information about treatments, send a self-addressed, business-sized envelope with 64¢ postage (in the US). Include a brief description of headache type and symptoms. A list of members in your state is also available on request.

National Institute of Mental Health. Office of Scientific Information, 5600 Fishers Lane, Parklawn Building, Room 7-103, Rockville, MD 20857. (301) 443-4513 (public inquiries branch). NIMH has free materials on mental health issues, including depression and psychological stress. They can't provide direct referral service, but they will refer people to professional organizations that can then provide a referral.

National Institute of Occupational Safety and Health (NIOSH). Technical Information Branch, Mail Stop C19, 4676 Columbia Parkway, Cincinnati, OH 45226. Information line: (800) 356-4674. NIOSH will provide information about seeking local assistance in occupational health issues, but they do not refer people directly to other agencies or services.

Office Technology Education Project. 1 Summer Street, Somerville, MA 02143. (617) 776-2777. Nonprofit organization that provides training, education, and information about the health implications and the social impact of new technologies.

Public Citizen Health Research Group. Washington, DC. (202) 833-3000. Every two years Public Citizen updates a list (organized by state) of doctors who have been disciplined by state boards. You can order the section for your state for about $10.

TCO (The Swedish Confederation of Professional Employees). 150 N. Michigan Avenue, Suite 1200, Chicago, IL 60601-7594. (312) 781-6223. Fax (312) 346-0683. Certifies equipment meeting its ergonomic and radiation standard for desktop computers. Offers book explaining monitor facts ($27). Sells kits to help evaluate monitors ($10) and software ($100 with disk).

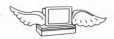

Newsletters & Magazines

■ ■ ■

CTDNews. 10 Railroad Avenue, PO Box 239, Haverford, PA 19041-0239. (800) 554-4283. Industry-oriented newsletter published 10 times a year reporting on cumulative trauma disorders (includes noncomputer sources). Source for legal, insurance, and regulatory information. Cost is $125 a year.

Managing Office Technology. 1100 Superior Avenue, Cleveland, OH 44114-2543. (216) 696-7000. Fax (216) 696-7658. Monthly publication that covers the integration of technology and human resources in the workplace.

Occupational Hazards Magazine. 1100 Superior Avenue, Cleveland, OH 44144-2543. (216) 696-7000. Fax (216) 696-7658. Monthly publication that covers occupational safety, health, industrial hygiene, and environmental management. Paid subscriptions are $45 per year or $5 per copy.

Occupational Health & Safety. PO Box 2573, 225 N. New Road, Waco, TX 76702-2573. (817) 776-9000. Fax (817) 776-9018. Magazine focuses on practical approaches for business to comply with OSHA, Department of Labor, NIOSH, and other regulatory agencies' guidelines, as well as information on voluntary guidelines, such as many ANSI standards.

VDT NEWS: The VDT Health and Safety Report. PO Box 1799, Grand Central Station, New York, NY 10163. (212) 517-2802. Fax (212) 734-0316. Particularly well-edited, in-depth newsletter that covers electromagnetic radiation, ergonomics, CTDs, and other health issues related to VDTs. Annual product directory included in subscription. Cost is $127 a year ($150 outside the United States).

Workplace Ergonomics. PO Box 2573, 225 N. New Road, Waco, TX 76702-2573. (817) 776-9000. Fax (817) 776-9018. Ergonomic issues in industrial and office settings, focusing on practical means for compliance.

RSI Network Newsletter. Grassroots electronic newsletter for people concerned about tendinitis, carpal tunnel syndrome, and other repetitive strain injuries. Available on many bulletin boards and on-line services. To subscribe via the Internet, send e-mail to: dadadata@world.std.com. Put "RSI Subscription" (without the quotes) in the "Subject:" line and you will be added to the distribution list.

Pointing Device Summary Document. Pete Johnson. Updated monthly on a Bitnet mailing list, C+Health. Subscribe by sending mail to the Internet mail address: listserv@iubvm.ucs.indiana.edu with the body of the message reading: "subscribe C+Health" followed by a space and then your first and last names (your e-mail address is automatically determined and should not be entered). If you have access to Usenet newsgroups, look for the group "bit.listserv.c+health".